D0908567

UNPLUGGED

Brian Mackenzie
Dr. Andy Galpin
& Phil White

Victory Belt Publishing

Las Vegas

First Published in 2017 by Victory Belt Publishing Inc.

ISBN 13: 978-1-628602-61-6

The information included in this book is for educational purposes only. It is not intended or implied to be a substitute for professional medical advice. The reader should always consult his or her health-care provider to determine the appropriateness of the information for his or her own situation or if he or she has any questions regarding a medical condition or treatment plan. Reading the information in this book does not create a physician-patient relationship.

Victory Belt® is a registered trademark of Victory Belt Publishing Inc.

Book design by Justin-Aaron Velasco
Illustrations by Justin-Aaron Velasco

Printed in CANADA
TC 0117

CONTENTS

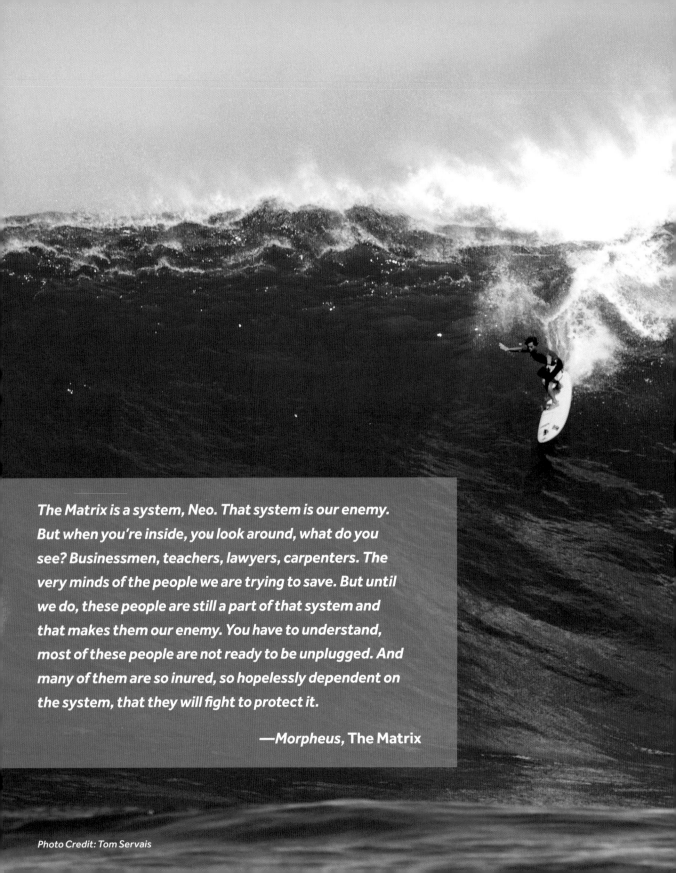

The Matrix is a system, Neo. That system is our enemy. But when you're inside, you look around, what do you see? Businessmen, teachers, lawyers, carpenters. The very minds of the people we are trying to save. But until we do, these people are still a part of that system and that makes them our enemy. You have to understand, most of these people are not ready to be unplugged. And many of them are so inured, so hopelessly dependent on the system, that they will fight to protect it.

—Morpheus, The Matrix

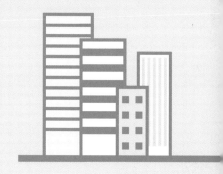

INTRODUCTION

Jerry Seinfeld once did a skit in which he imagined aliens looking down from space, seeing us scooping up our dogs' poop, and assuming that it was our pets who were the real masters. Ten years on, what would extraterrestrials deduce if they observed us running around following the commands of little devices on our wrists and checking these tiny screens obsessively every few minutes? They'd likely conclude that some all-powerful overlord was telling us what to do at all times through these strange gadgets. This isn't the stuff of science fiction or a stand-up comedy routine but a daily reality for the millions of people who've made fitness wearables and apps a multibillion-dollar industry.

In early human societies, physical prowess was a survival tool. Our ancestors needed to be able to fend off and outrun predators and hunt and kill their own prey to stay alive and feed themselves and their families. As we progressed and started living in more-sophisticated tribes, the need for speed, strength, power, and endurance remained practical, as people had to be able to fight and ultimately defeat rival groups. Many ancient cultures also had physically demanding rites of passage that people had to undertake to confirm their transition into adulthood.

Such instincts were also directed toward athletic competitions that determined who could lift and throw the most weight and run the fastest. While the ancient Greeks and Romans maintained formidable armies for fighting off their enemies, they also staged sporting contests for the sake of ego and amusement: the ancient Olympic Games, gladiator contests, and so on. The Middle Ages saw knights jousting and strongman cultures developing in countries like Scotland (whose stone-lifting-and-throwing traditions would evolve into the modern Highland Games) and the Basque region of Spain.

Fast-forward a few hundred years to the late 1800s and reductions in working hours birthed a relatively new concept: leisure. With industrialization, people began to have more money to do things outside of the workplace and more time to participate in and watch sports. Soccer, baseball, football, rugby, and the modern Olympics resulted.

But even the most visionary Victorians could never have imagined the extent to which recreation would grow from spending a nice afternoon kicking a ball around a field or paying to watch their favorite team do so into a multibillion-dollar global sports and fitness industry. They certainly couldn't have anticipated that active leisure would eventually move indoors, that the penny-farthing bicycles that one pedaled precariously around the village square would be replaced by rows of stationary bicycles that display virtual maps, heart rate, and power output. That the humble pocket

BRIAN MACKENZIE, DR. ANDY GALPIN & PHIL WHITE

watch used to time men and horses as they ran around tracks would evolve into powerful, "smart" devices capable of capturing gigabytes of biometric data. Or that we'd somehow go from drinking a pint of "Good for You" Guinness with friends in a pub after a long walk in the countryside to ingesting a daily cocktail of chemicals designed to yield maximum results from a strictly regimented training program.

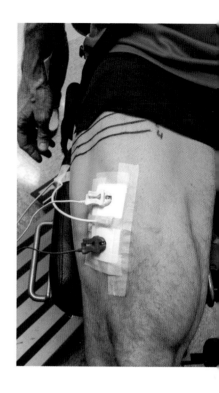

Leisure was initially available only to the rich, as their diminished need for physical work (working in the fields, building houses, and so on) afforded them the extra time to expend physical energy in sport. What they didn't see coming was the next major change in society, heralded by the advent of the personal computer. In fact, they certainly couldn't have predicted the speed at which our society would reach nearly complete automation, meaning that the physicality of most jobs has been all but eliminated. Although we're not quite there, Moore's law—which notes that the number of transistors per inch on a circuit doubles every year, with corresponding increases in computing power—suggests we're shockingly closer to that reality than most accept.

Thus, we're at the dawn of a new age in which physical exertion is almost completely removed from our daily lives, a gap that we try to fill with technology-dictated exercise. The major difference between the late-Victorian-era shift away from physical activity and the current one is speed. The need for nonwork physical activity during the Industrial Revolution took decades to fully manifest itself, giving individuals and society as a whole time to adjust so that no major decreases in human health occurred. However, the New Industrial Revolution is happening in the blink of a species' eye.

We need to adjust. Now.

The push for everyone to take ten thousand steps a day was an early fix, and while this may return us to a base level of physical activity (in other words, simulating the movement that used to be part of everyone's working day) to help stop us from dying from preventable, chronic lifestyle diseases, it won't suffice to fully eliminate the burden of a sedentary life.

Technology companies got wind of our culture's sedentary lifestyle–related issues and are pouring billions of dollars into fitness trackers to help return us to a minimal level of physical activity. Some even aim to improve the peak performance of the elite.

Some people view such changes as progress, and indeed, technology publications and sports scientists alike are touting the benefits of Big Data and the journey toward "the quantified self." Companies are certainly happy to take the money that we're all too ready to hand over for fitness wearables, sensor-equipped shoes and clothing, and an endless array of supplements. But their profit is our loss. Individually and collectively, we've forgotten what it means to enjoy playing, experimenting, and expressing our humanity in fully engaged exertion.

Scott Adams, creator of the *Dilbert* comic strip that has long lampooned overdependence on technology, cautions,

> All of your autonomy is going away. Suppose you had a fitness band five or ten years from now and it tells you when to take a sip of water, and can tell you what kind of food you should eat and when and tells you when you should sleep. In the beginning you're going to say, "Oh, good suggestion. I'll either do that or not." But eventually you're going to see that its suggestion is better than whatever you would've done on your own. You're just going to start following that app, and eventually it's going to be completely controlling your life, while you have the sensation that you're deciding.[1]

Adams and other critics of the self-quantification movement see that our phones, watches, and wearables promise insight, knowledge, and freedom, but what they really deliver is information overload, confusion, and servitude. In spending our so-called leisure time indoors mindlessly pounding away on stationary objects, we're severing our connection to the natural world. As my good friend and surfer Laird Hamilton told me, "Technology's tendency to insulate us from nature while we're participating in it ultimately leads to us failing to absorb all it has to offer. We're missing out because we're looking down at our phones the whole time, and that's having an effect on our brain."[2]

With our ever-increasing dependence on technology, we're outsourcing our independence, and we risk creating a dangerous addiction that can wreak physical, emotional, and societal havoc. And while we waste hours artificially stimulating our brains with gadgets in our homes, gyms, and fitness studios, we're depriving ourselves of the exposure to wind, sunlight, water, and the other elements that can help us be fully alive, if only we'd let them.

Those of us who do make the effort to be active outside are little better off. With headphones blocking out birdsong, sunglasses and sunscreen shielding us from the light we've somehow come to fear, and gizmos in our pockets and on our wrists diverting our attention, we've turned rich-tasting experiences into dried-out, flavorless husks that exist only to

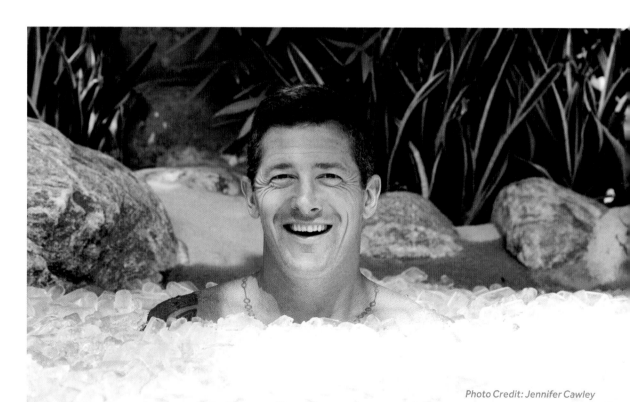

Photo Credit: Jennifer Cawley

provide us with a few more steps on our activity tracker and a couple more ounces lost when we step on our digital scale. As we relentlessly work toward our goals, we lose awareness of anything beyond what's right in front of us and neglect to do what my friend Tim Ferriss suggests and "pause occasionally to appreciate the little things, like meaningless beauty that has nothing to do with any objective, nothing to do with any metric, and nothing to do with any plan."[3]

Even as we're losing our ability to wonder at the sun rising above the sea or setting behind a mountain, we're focusing more and more on material gain. We mistakenly believe that dropping thousands of dollars on ultralight bike frames, custom-made paddleboards, and other high-priced gear will improve our performance and fulfill our materialistic urges, when in reality it has just created an unwinnable arms race that's sucking away what's left of our souls.

From recreational sports leagues to the pros to youth sports, we've abandoned spontaneous, chaotic, and unbound exploration for a predictable, controllable, regimented grind that does little to satisfy beyond the narrow, self-limiting goals we set for ourselves. And the programs that we adhere to so religiously and that tell us what to do, how much, and when are largely based on outdated notions and popularly accepted junk science concepts that mislead us yet further.

As a result, we burn ourselves out mentally and wear our bodies down physically, until we lapse back into our old bad lifestyle habits in search of solace. Despite the promises of technology, we're sicker, more worried, and less fulfilled than ever before. Indeed, 2016 saw the first reduction in life expectancy in the US in decades.[4] This came despite the fact that as much as two-thirds of all health-care expenditures— which continue to skyrocket—is on new technologies that promise to make us healthier and cure us quicker.[5]

So why is our overdependence on fitness technology a problem? First, we've distanced ourselves from nature to the point that we barely even notice the world around us, let alone allow ourselves the physical, mental, and emotional benefits that regular, unfiltered immersion in it can provide. Second, we're sacrificing genuine, deep interactions with real humans for the artificial community that online apps provide. And third, we've stopped listening to the innate instincts that our body provides, preferring to be semiconscious and outsource decision-making to technology that is often wildly inaccurate. Instead of wielding fitness technology to solve problems, increase self-education, and enhance our connection to ourselves, other people, and the world around us, we've allowed it to create new issues, dull our understanding, and isolate us. In our blind belief that more technology equals advancement, we're arguably regressing.

Then there's the fact that despite all the gaudy marketing claims of fitness technology, our performance hasn't actually improved much with all this gear, if at all. When exercise scientists put Olympic one-hundred-meter silver medalist Andre De Grasse in the same clothing and shoes that Jesse Owens wore in 1936 and had him run on cinders instead of a modern synthetic track, his best time was actually *slower* than the man who famously defied Hitler in the 1936 Olympics. And if we look at weightlifting feats, today's tech-aided power athletes might be setting new squat and dead lift records but are lagging far behind the stone-lifting and object-throwing feats of predecessors from hundreds of years ago (see Chris McDougall's excellent book *Natural Born Heroes* for examples). We've been misled into believing that working out endlessly indoors in $200 shoes under the guidance of wearable algorithms will somehow transform us from Tony Stark into Iron Man. But once we take off the flying suit, we find we're just as fallible and fragile as ever. Or we try to simplify and isolate elements of the incredibly complex human organism and start measuring the wrong things or things that cannot be accurately quantified.

According to an Ericsson ConsumerLab report entitled "Wearable Technology and the Internet of Things," sales of wearables almost doubled in the past year.[6] Without a doubt, some people claim to love having a device on their wrist 24/7, but for many others, the sheen has worn off. One survey reported that 79 percent of people who used a popular device felt pressured to reach their daily targets, with 59 percent saying it controlled their daily routines and 30 percent viewing it as their enemy.[7] Others claim that their wearable inaccurately measured their heart rates, and they are so upset about this that they've filed lawsuits.[8] While this might be going a little far, there is evidence to support their claims: multiple studies have found that activity trackers' heart rate monitoring is only 80 percent accurate with higher heart rates.[9] Regardless of how such legal proceedings pan out, it's fair to say that we're putting too much faith in wearable technology and have become far too dependent on constant body monitoring, introducing a new source of stress into the very physical activity that's meant to relax us.

If you wear a device 24/7, you begin relying on it to tell you how your body is performing, what you're doing right and wrong, and how much effort you're putting in. It used to be that we'd listen to our own instincts about such things and act accordingly. But now millions of people are content to hand over their self-monitoring and decision-making to a machine, which, they reason, must know better because it's "smart" technology. Tim Ferriss told me, "Technology is an excellent tool and a terrible master."[10]

When we submit to this artificial master's orders, we abandon not only our decision-making but also the spontaneity that puts the fun in physical activity. In December 2016, waterman wunderkind Kai Lenny shocked the surfing world when he pulled off an unprecedented air grab at Hawaii's Peahi break, which is so formidable that it has earned the nickname "Jaws." There was no piece of fitness technology that could've conceived the maneuver, let alone given Kai the instructions to pull it off on a wave face taller than your house. Instead, he relied on the intuition he had honed during thousands of hours in the water.

"I didn't go into that wave thinking, 'I'm going to down the line, do a giant air, grab the rail and tweak it out,'" Kai told me.

> It was all instinctual and in the moment. When I towed in I recognized it wasn't the biggest wave of the day and was like, "Okay I'm going to fade, and then I'm going to come back." As I went into my bottom turn, I was setting up and thought, "There's a good little chip shot here." Then I hit the bump and got all this projection into the air. I learned from kitesurfing that by overexaggerating the maneuver it gives yourself time in the air, whereas if you just stop you usually fall. I was slowly tweaking my board out more and more as it went higher, and then as it was coming down, I started to reverse that and was bringing it in. Right when I landed I let go of the rail, and then just naturally went into how I would land any trick when I'm kitesurfing. I did a little chop hump back down the wave and then kicked out.[11]

Such creativity and innovation is possible only when we allow ourselves to fully focus on a singular experience, engaging all our senses. And yet all too many of us are preventing this by enabling our fitness technology to dictate how we move, when, and for how long. Then we further remove the conditions needed for improvisation by putting ourselves in restricted indoor settings that do little to challenge or inspire. Maybe we won't ever land an air grab at Jaws, carve fresh powder down an Alaskan peak, or huck a one-hundred-foot waterfall, but we're cutting off the path to whatever our greatest athletic achievements could be by settling for tech-imposed limitations.

Perhaps only a fool would attempt to urge the masses to abandon technology and return to their roots. Those who don't embrace change usually get crushed faster than a newbie surfer being swallowed by a one-hundred-foot wave. The real issue is not the technology itself but our misconception of what it can or will do for us, refusal to accept its limitations, and fixation on fitness tracking, which deadens our senses.

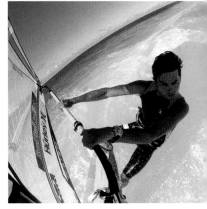

Photo Credit: Kai Lenny

It's time to stop, take a breath, and hit a big reset button. We need to sit up, take notice, and recognize that these tools can be either a help or a hindrance. The key to using them more safely, discriminately, and productively is to understand what we're working toward and how we can use technology to help us get there. Unfortunately, most fall into the trap of thinking that a higher score on their wearable or achieving a personal-best race time is the end goal. Then we put our full trust in our wrist-worn autopilot to get us there, not realizing that the time will come when we'll need to take the controls and fly the plane ourselves—or not acknowledging that all too often the gauges we're reading to check our progress not only are faulty but also can take us way off our intended course. It took years of unsatisfying racing and countless injuries for me to figure this out. The same happened to Andy.

He once had the opportunity to train under legendary American weight lifter Tommy Kono. As it was early in Andy's career, he was eager to extract every possible pearl of wisdom from the former Olympian. So he asked Kono how his positioning looked after nearly every repetition. Kono refused to answer this misguided question and replaced it with a better one: "How did it feel?"

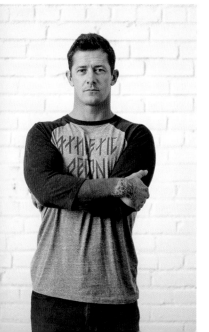

Hi, this is Brian Mackenzie, performance specialist, founder of Power Speed Endurance, and cofounder of XPT Life. For the sake of clarity, my coauthors and I have written this book in the first person from my perspective. And speaking of those coauthors, they are Dr. Andy Galpin, professor of kinesiology at the Center for Sport Performance at California State University, Fullerton, host of the *Body of Knowledge* podcast, and secret weapon of dozens of pro athletes and Olympians, and Phil White, coauthor of *Waterman 2.0* and *Flight Plan* with Dr. Kelly Starrett and *Game Changer* with Fergus Connolly.

The problem was that Andy had yet to comprehend two important concepts. First, quality is preeminent. Whether optimal health or peak performance is the goal, better movement always equals better output and fewer injuries. And second, feeling is understanding. Beginners often lack calibration, knowledge, and awareness of the factors that are key to movement success. Technology can exponentially speed up this learning curve. However, if the perfect movement cannot be replicated when the technology is eliminated entirely, the user lacks true understanding and does not truly own the movement.

The gold standard—which, for many of the athletes I work with, is a gold *medal* standard—is being able to recognize and correct movement errors with *only* your own feelings. Continual reliance on technology eliminates the user's opportunity to transition from the beginner to intermediate levels, or, if they're already there, from intermediate to advanced.

Another issue is that, while a technology can solve a specific problem, its use can also unleash some unintended consequences that can prove harmful. Take soap as an example. Washing our hands helps prevent the spread of everyday ailments like the common cold, removes dirt and grime, and even stems the proliferation of deadly viruses like Ebola. But in an attempt to supposedly improve soap by adding antibacterial agents, manufacturers started a cascade that has culminated in the rise of so-called superbugs and resistant pathogens that no antibiotic can cure (to say nothing of the overprescription of antibiotics, which is exacerbating the issue). We inevitably miss more than we see, and we're likely using technology today that will have a negative impact that doesn't manifest itself until sometime in the future, when we've increased our understanding.

This is why we're not saying that we're against fitness technology or that you should stop using it completely— technology *can* solve problems—but rather that you should take a more careful approach to how you use it, when, and why. While many people are going too far in allowing devices to dictate their actions and thinking, it's also possible to go too far the other way. In the movie *Captain Fantastic*, Viggo Mortensen's character tries to go off the grid and raise his kids in the forests of Washington State. He soon realizes that, though he still wants to teach his children to connect with nature and be self-reliant, a halfway solution is more realistic. Even the high priest of naturalism, Henry David Thoreau, came to believe that he had to reenter society after his isolation experience, which led to the profound insights he detailed in *Walden*.

That's why our goal isn't to tell you to move out into the woods, dig a survival shelter, and shun technology completely, but rather to guide you to elevated self-awareness and equip you with the tools to use wearables, quantification, and testing more appropriately. By the time you finish reading this book, we want to have liberated you from dependence on fitness technology, reintroduced you to the endless possibilities of outdoor activity, and helped you find better ways to use your devices to heighten your consciousness, instead of allowing them to be dominating taskmasters. In the following pages, we'll help everyone from the elite coach to the competitive athlete to the everyday exerciser learn to use technology as a calibration tool to expand their awareness (and thus, true understanding) of high-quality, efficient, and powerful human movement. Along the way, we'll introduce you to some simple, evidence-based steps you can take to improve not just your fitness but also your overall health and well-being. Reading *Unplugged* will enable you to:

- Understand the value and limitations of technology for athletic performance, fitness, health, and lifestyle
- Know how and when to utilize physical activity technologies in your everyday life—and when not to
- Avoid the common mistakes most people make with wearables and tracking apps
- Understand which technologies are most effective and which are a waste of money

Once you've reached this level of understanding, we'll show you how to:

- End your addiction to fitness technology and start using it as a tool for cueing, learning, and sensing instead of a crutch
- Stop obsessively quantifying your training and focus on the quality of it instead
- Improve self-awareness and increase self-reliance
- Break the stress cycle that constant monitoring exacerbates
- Reconnect with nature by spending less time indoors and more outside
- Revitalize your senses by ditching wearables when you're outdoors
- Use technology to link what you're feeling to what's going on in your body and how you should respond
- Upgrade virtual competition and training to real community
- Rediscover the value of coaches' expertise, curation, and intuition, which can't be replaced by technology
- Cultivate physical practices that are refreshing and restorative instead of draining
- Take back control of your health, fitness, and performance

This is not some Luddite fantasy where we're going to collect all our fitness wearables and smartphones, throw them onto a bonfire, and dance around it. Nor am I saying that you should never set foot in a gym again. And I promise that I'm not some hippie who's proposing that you go off the grid and start living off the land! Instead, I hope that this book will help you to become less fixated on technology, more engaged with the outside world, and more aware of yourself, to the good of your health.

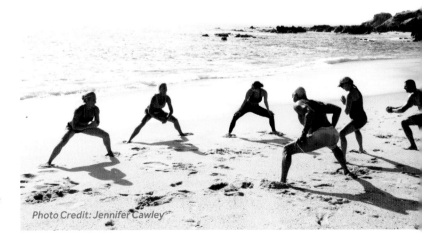

Photo Credit: Jennifer Cawley

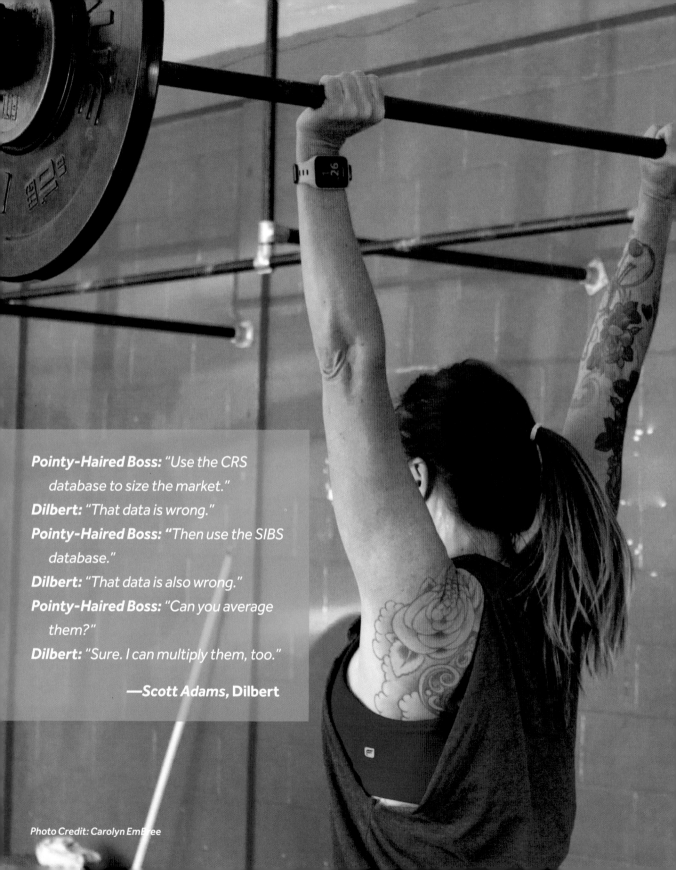

Pointy-Haired Boss: *"Use the CRS database to size the market."*
Dilbert: *"That data is wrong."*
Pointy-Haired Boss: *"Then use the SIBS database."*
Dilbert: *"That data is also wrong."*
Pointy-Haired Boss: *"Can you average them?"*
Dilbert: *"Sure. I can multiply them, too."*

—*Scott Adams,* **Dilbert**

Photo Credit: Carolyn EmBree

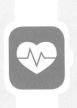

CHAPTER 1
THE WEARABLES REVOLUTION: MAKING SENSE OF MEASURABLES

In the first quarter of 2016 alone, Americans bought 19.7 million wearables, an increase of 67 percent from the start of 2015. Later in the year, the market leader's European sales increased 64 percent. By 2020, the global market for fitness-focused apps and devices is expected to grow to over $30 billion.[12] This means that more than ever, we're looking at our wrists not only to check the time but also to see how much we've moved, what our heart rate is doing, and how we're stacking up against yesterday's tallies. Why make the effort to be conscious of your activity when you can delegate the task to an ever-willing, always-on device? But while it might seem easier to just let technology decide, there are some pitfalls to doing so.

The Downsides of Wearables

The appeal of wearables seems self-evident: all that data at your fingertips, reminders and rewards to help motivate you, automated programs with milestones to help you reach your goals. The downsides, unfortunately, are less obvious, but they're no less real. Yes, wearables help motivate us at first, but what happens when the initial enthusiasm they spark wears off? And yes, it's handy to have a device that tells us what to do and when, but what does that do to our self-awareness and knowledge of our bodies? We're making trade-offs that we may not even be aware of.

Wearing Your Heart on Your Sleeve

For people who want to transform their sedentary lifestyle into an active one and don't know where to start, a wearable can provide some early motivation and accountability. Buying such a device, or a fitness app for a phone or watch, can also have the benefit of changing movement from an afterthought to a daily priority. But we know that good intentions are one thing and sticking to them another. Ninety-two percent of people discard their New Year's resolutions by March 1, which is why gyms that are crowded in January are half-empty two months later.[13] It's the same with pledges of "I'm going to get in shape" made any time of year. We start off full of enthusiasm, which a wearable can help encourage, but soon backslide once our progress stagnates, or we fall back on one of the old excuses, like "I just have bad genes" or "I'm too busy." One study found that 50 percent of people who buy a wearable stop using it within six months.[14] If it was their sole source of motivation, their new healthy lifestyle soon falls by the wayside, too.

One of the issues here is that when we introduce technology into the mix, it begins to change the way that we trigger the release of neurotransmitters. If you've ever experienced the so-called runner's high or a more profound sense of pleasure when you're doing something active, it's partly because your brain is prompting the release of "happy" hormones. This is one of the reasons that exercise can be habit-forming in a good way—we crave that shot of dopamine and other chemicals that give us the natural high.

In a perfect, unplugged world, we'd just enjoy fun activities in their purest form and be content to reap the rewards that they provide. Yet all too often we try to enhance our experiences with an app or wearable, not realizing that doing so changes the source of our habit-reward system. Every time you look down to check your heart rate, pace, or split time, your brain gives you a little dopamine hit. In an article for *Psychology Today*, Dr. Susan Weinschenk writes, "The dopamine system is most powerfully stimulated when the information coming in is small so that it doesn't fully satisfy. A short text or tweet (can only be 140 characters!) is ideally suited to send your dopamine system raging."[15] The same is true of the momentary information you get by looking at your app, hearing a virtual coach shout encouragement in your ear, or even checking a text or e-mail on your smartwatch. Before you know it, you're looking at your device more and more to get your fix, and the activity itself becomes secondary.

Yet at a certain point, even the biggest dopamine junkies find that technology is no longer satisfying their insatiable craving for more and more neurochemicals. Or they look at the data and find that they're failing to meet their goals. And so, despite the compulsion to keep the device on their wrist, in their ears, or in their pockets, they cast it aside. Because their motivation was coming from an external source, removing it means that many struggle to keep being active. A Duke University study found that as a result, "those who had quit tracking ended up doing less of their given activity than the people who'd never had any numbers attached to it in the first place."[16]

So what can you do if you've quit fitness tracking and are struggling with motivation? One answer lies in hacking your neurobiology by getting into the flow states (heightened periods of total engagement that elevate cognitive and kinesthetic performance) that Steven Kotler explores in *The Rise of Superman*. Taking on a physical challenge that pushes your ability, requires complete concentration, and eliminates all outside distractions not only leads to the physical performance leaps that flow makes possible but also offers a deep and lasting sense of satisfaction. The athletes Steven profiles—including such game changers as Jeremy Jones and Danny Way—are not motivated by tangible rewards like trophies or external motivation from a fitness tracker, but rather by a desire to push both their own boundaries and those of their sports. From a brain chemistry standpoint, flow provides all the feel-good benefits of a dopamine shot and many more. Check out the last chapter of this book for Steven's tips on how to access this elevated state and its benefits (even if you're not planning to jump the Great Wall of China on a skateboard, like Danny Way).

Know Thyself

Adherence is just one of the issues with wearables. To me, an even bigger problem is that by connecting yet another area of our life to technology, we're pushing ever further from really knowing ourselves and interacting in an unfiltered, authentic way with our natural environment. In this age of distraction, we're also adding just another layer to the issue of continuous partial attention, whereby we never fully focus on one thing at a time. We already had a device that intruded on our work productivity, our time with friends and family, and our recreation, and now, with the rise of wearables, many people are hijacked by two or three. This means our attention spans are even shorter and we're more distracted than ever.

As a result, we're losing our ability to be conscious of what we're doing, how we're feeling, and what's going on around us. This is bad enough in a gym, but it's when we get outside that the constant checking of a tiny screen truly wreaks havoc, downgrading what should be a rich, elemental, and sensory experience into yet another task we need to complete to meet our daily goals for steps taken and calories burned. And if we fail to achieve these algorithm-imposed goals, we feel inadequate and worthless. So while wearables might be beneficial to get some people on the road to better health, for many of us they've worn out their welcome.

Pace Yourself

One of the most common ways that recreational athletes use wearables and apps is to pace themselves for training sessions, whether that's per lap when running, per mile when cycling, or per five hundred meters when rowing. We've come to believe that to stick to a training program, we've got to maintain a certain pace, and that we can't do this ourselves. So we rely on a device to do it for us. But this assumption is wrong.

A few years ago, Andy conducted a study that required a sample group of cross-country competitors to run eight thousand meters at a comfortable pace. They weren't allowed to use any technology—not even an analog watch. Three

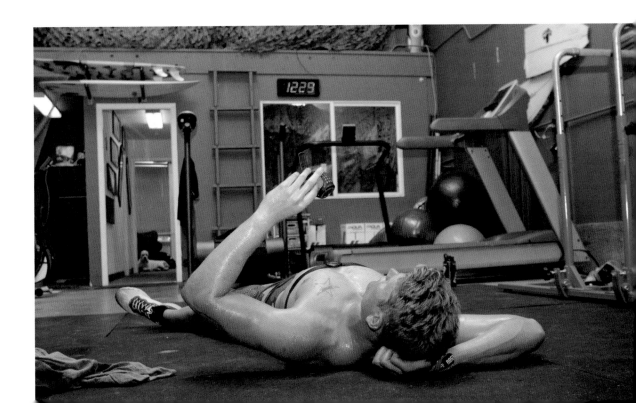

weeks later they were asked to repeat the distance with the same amount of effort, with the only guidance being to focus on how it felt to run at the same pace as during the first test. Remarkably, all the runners' finishing times were within two seconds of their original times. This suggests that we're far more capable of self-regulating pace and effort level than we give ourselves credit for—if only we can stop relying on our technology and start trusting our innate ability.

The best way to apply this to a training program is to use a simple device to measure your workouts for the first three to four weeks and make notes after each session about how it felt. You could even gauge your effort level on a scale from one to ten, with ten being the max. Then review both your progress and these notes. Your goal should always be continual, gradual progression, so as long as you're not feeling completely burned out, keep doing the program while aiming for similar exertion and feelings in each session, setting aside your technology. After another four weeks, retest yourself to calibrate where you're at. But if you're regressing, plateauing, or just destroying yourself, then back off the intensity or duration a bit, with the simple aim of taking it a bit easier in each workout. You might find that you're not pushing hard enough, so you need to dial it up. In this second four-week phase, use your intuition to guide you and utilize technology sparingly to assess, inform, and recalibrate as needed.

Drowning in Data

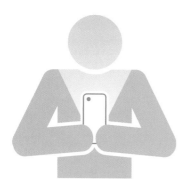

Big Data—aka the drive to collect as much information as possible—might work for a multinational company like Walmart or Amazon that's tracking metrics on millions of products in real time. But it isn't applicable in the same way to human performance, no matter what the prophets of self-quantification proclaim. A single metric could be a big deal in lots of areas of life, from the temperature in the weather forecast to the pressure in your car's tires to the price of a company's stock. But because the human body is an incredibly complex system of systems, looking at just one data point from a single aspect of our biology—like heart rate—and using it to make blanket recommendations for how you should tailor your entire training program is extremely foolish. And yet that's precisely what millions of people are letting their activity trackers and apps do.

If you're going to monitor your body, it's a far better idea to collect multiple data points over an extended period of time, like a week or a month, and then share it with a trusted coach who can use her knowledge to help make sense of it and dig into how you perform when certain numbers are up or down. She can then make more informed recommendations for your overall lifestyle—from activity to nutrition to recovery—than a device is ever going to come up with.

We can think of the issues with data as falling into two categories: problems with applicability (not all data is useful) and problems with accuracy (devices can be inaccurate).

Confusing Information for Insight

How much of the information we're collecting about ourselves is truly usable for improving performance? One manufacturer of a sensor-equipped tennis racket that sends data on topspin and backspin, serve speed, and more to a phone app in real time promises that you can "know more about your game to better perform." Is this really the case, or will you simply have more information?

If a tennis player is going to work with a coach who knows which numbers are relevant to a certain facet of their game and indicate opportunities for improvement, then that's fine. But there's the danger of confusing measurements for outcomes. Say the app told you that your first serve in a match averaged eighty-nine miles per hour, which was down 10 percent from the previous round of a tournament. You could take this to mean that you needed to go out and fire a couple of hundred serves before facing your next opponent. Or maybe you'd assume that your serving arm was too weak, so you'd better get in a hard weights session to top up your strength. Both deductions could lead to actions that harm your play in the next match, and both are completely arbitrary. Also, say that in that match, you prevented your opponent from breaking your serve. While the speed was down, maybe the accuracy went up. And maybe you were serving into a headwind for two sets, which reduced your average speed. So that first-serve average, though below par, was more than enough to get the job done.

This is an example of trying to draw meaningful conclusions from data points without taking quality or outcome (did you win or lose?) into account. Another risk with relying on numbers to inform your training is that they almost always reduce performance to speed, power, and strength. This overlooks the fact that your expression of all these physical qualities is limited by your skill level, which everyone, from novices to world champions, should always be working to improve. In addition, supposedly smart technology doesn't take into account strategy or tactics, or the mental and emotional components of performance, which are just as important as physical ones. Just because we're measuring more doesn't mean we have greater understanding. So we should either stop using fitness trackers, restrict them to the role of coaching aids, or use them to monitor our progress over time, rather than allowing them to dictate day-to-day strategy.

Those who do rely on metrics to dictate their every move are making a simple error. If we outsource our consciousness to a machine, we come to think that data is understanding. It's not. Rather, data is knowledge that requires interpretation to be applicable. This is a fancy way of saying that yes, data can be helpful, but decades of experience on the part of the athlete and coach are needed to fully understand what it's saying and how to use it to solve problems. Context is critical if data is to be applied correctly. So the next time you sit down to study the metrics from a workout, consider whether you truly comprehend what that day's data is telling you when compared to similar information from the previous week,

The Scientist and the Practitioner

For a long time there has been a gap between what science tells us and how coaches and performance specialists put these findings into practice. There's also the issue that only study authors and journal editors actually read up to half of all academic papers, which suggests that only fellow scientists can make sense of the geek speak.[17] This is why Andy is committed to writing for the layperson, particularly the coaching community. A big part of his mission and mine is closing the researcher-practitioner gap so we can figure out which measurables are meaningful and what we should do with them in designing evidence-based programs for our athletes. Such programming will use wearables and other technology appropriately as tools, rather than cutting out coaching expertise and deferring to an algorithm devised in a Silicon Valley hipster coffee shop.

month, or year. If you don't know and haven't the first clue how to use it productively to improve your performance, you either need to call in a coach or stop tracking this data point.

Getting to Grips with Genetic Testing

What if you could not only look inside your own body to see how it functions but actually peek inside your DNA to discover your genetic performance potential? Such insight is exactly what several companies are now offering. They promise to tell you how well your body absorbs certain nutrients, your muscle fiber composition (slow-twitch versus fast-twitch), and how well you respond to different types of energy system–based training, such as anaerobic or aerobic.

The question is what you should make of the results. If you find that you have a high percentage of fast-twitch muscle fibers, should this encourage you to start playing an explosive sport like basketball and doing lots of Olympic lifting and

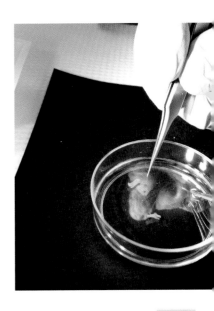

plyometrics because of your genetic predisposition to this type of training? Or, since you're already a natural at such things, should you work on developing your slow-twitch muscle fibers because your DNA has disadvantaged you in this area? The same goes for energy systems. If you're an aerobic responder, should you start signing up for marathons or triathlons and gearing all your preparation around such events? Or is it better to concentrate on overcoming your anaerobic weaknesses?

Similar quandaries await in nutrition. Nutrient levels vary daily and are a moving target, so it's hard to get definitive answers about what you're getting too much of and what you're lacking from a one-off test. Nutrient absorption is impacted not just by genetics but also by the timing and dosage of other substances, not to mention sleep, stress levels, and exertion. The same goes for hormone balance, which can be altered by sex, sickness, and any number of other variables.

The reality is that while genetic testing holds a lot of promise, it's still in its infancy and you're better off saving your money. There just isn't a large enough sample size currently in the databases of the testing companies, hospitals, or government agencies to draw meaningful conclusions. It's also worth noting that no gene has but a single function; each is involved in hundreds or even thousands of bodily processes. Every gene also interacts with one another in ways we cannot yet understand. So it's an oversimplification to say, "Well, gene X is turned on, so you should do Y in your training from now on."

We also need to think carefully about the motivations of genetic testing organizations. These may well be noble, but let's be honest. They're for-profit companies who stand to gain a lot for giving you a little information that's hazy at best. When you sign up, they get all your data points, which they add to the information they've already harvested, helping them to become more accurate. In return, you get some nice, colorful graphics depicting certain levels and a few prescriptions for what to eat, how to train, and so on. Amazon had a similar motivation when it purchased the power-reader website Goodreads. Is it just a coincidence that many of the testing providers also sell higher-priced training and nutrition packages? This isn't altruism. It's commercialism!

So is there a place for testing? Absolutely. But you should only have a doctor scan for major diseases and do the usual bloodwork in annual checkups. Then, if you want to, do cheap assessments on your grip strength, VO_2 max, or lean body mass, which are well understood and are the main predictors of long life or early mortality. Other, more progressive assessments (particularly genetic testing) might well yield useful insights in the near future, as the field of genomics continues advancing rapidly, but for right now their cost outweighs their utility.

What's Your Problem?

One advantage that genetic testing could provide is to identify how genes contribute to issues that affect some people but aren't a nationwide problem. Let's take our biggest addiction, caffeine. If you can drink a latte at 8 p.m. and still sleep fine, you're likely a fast metabolizer of caffeine. If that latte would keep you up until 3 a.m., you're probably a slow metabolizer. People whose bodies can process caffeine more quickly can typically drink five to eight cups a day with few, if any, ill effects. But studies show that for slow caffeine metabolizers, such a high intake can increase their chances of developing heart disease.[18]

We sometimes make assumptions about how we handle caffeine or other foods, but we don't really know for sure. Genetic testing can remove the guesswork and let us know how quickly we metabolize certain substances and what the health consequences could be. We could then make more informed lifestyle adjustments to improve our well-being and reduce certain health risks.

Admitting the Limitations of the Quantified Self

Read enough geeky magazines and you'll see that some technology prophets and their disciples think that in our (read: their) infinite wisdom, we can use fitness trackers, apps, and smartwatches to monitor every aspect of our biology and then use the data to make our lives into some kind of überhealthy utopia. In Dave Eggers's *The Circle,* the creator of the book's social media system states, "I'm a believer in the perfectibility of human beings."

This kind of statement is just vain hubris. Yet it's not much of an exaggeration of the attitude that prevails in the fitness tech community. The trouble is that for all their fancy speeches and I-want-that gadgets, people with this mind-set are failing to acknowledge the reality that there's far more about the body and brain that we don't know than we're letting on. And, sorry to burst the bubble, this isn't going to change anytime soon. The thousands of processes that are occurring within each of us in every microsecond are incredibly complex, and each is tied in to the others in ways that we cannot hope to ever fully understand. So while the term "the quantified self" might be here to stay, it implies a notion of perfectibility that's impossible to achieve, which means it will remain nothing more than a hollow buzzword. And if we keep chasing performance simply for the sake of improving our numbers, we're missing out on the fun of being active.

No Good Answers to a Bad Question

One of the latest trends in the wearables space is the use of "smart clothing." This uses embedded sensors to measure certain things about our bodies. Some just replicate the functions of wrist-worn devices, measuring heart rate, steps taken, and so on. But other manufacturers are attempting to quantify elements of performance, such as muscle recruitment: at least a couple of these companies' product lines measure the activation of various muscle groups during a given exercise and then make recommendations on what you need to do differently to better engage those that aren't pulling their weight. The trouble is, who's to say what percentage of quad, glute, or hamstring activation you should ideally have in a squat or a dead lift? This is completely arbitrary, as is the subsequent advice for supposed improvements. Then there's the fact that measuring muscle activation and recruitment on the surface of the skin is inaccurate and error-prone. So maybe that smart clothing isn't quite as clever as its makers think it is. Rather, it's giving you information that the information is arbitrary, not personalized, or both.

Say that you're an injured basketball player and you start using a pair of smart, sensor-embedded shorts to measure your glute activation during a certain rehab exercise. If learning which variation of this exercise better activates your glutes gets you back on the basketball court five days earlier than expected, then perhaps you should keep using the shorts. If not, then it'd be better for you to set this $700 item aside and instead defer to the expertise of your physical therapist, who may well be able to identify and correct your issue (in this case, your glutes not firing enough) just by looking at how you move.

How Many Calories Did You Burn?

A January 2017 study published in the journal *Medicine and Science in Sport and Exercise* compared multiple consumer-level activity trackers to a more expensive calorimeter to see how accurately they measured calories burned during walking, running, cycling outside, and pedaling on an exercise bike. The researchers found that the commercially available devices varied wildly. One device was 92 percent accurate for walking and running but managed just 40.4 percent accuracy for outdoor cycling and registered a donut—0 percent!—for cycling on a stationary bike.[19] So if you're a walker or runner, such a wearable would just about do its job, if you're okay with that 8 percent error margin. But what cyclist in their right mind

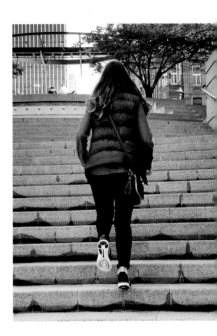

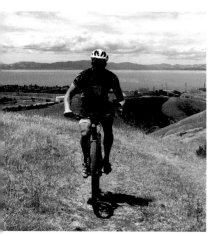

Photo Credit: Patrick Cummins

would want to rely on a device that's only 40 percent accurate if they're on a road or mountain bike and completely inaccurate if they're training indoors? Nobody. Yet millions of cyclists do put their faith in their trackers and, in fact, are arguably the most hard-core self-quantification demographic.

And they're not the only ones looking to count calories. Certain fitness programs want participants to hit a certain calorie number on rowing machines before they move on to the next activity, while a big part of the entire jogging movement was calorie burning. The entire diet industry is obsessed with both sides of the equation—calories in and calories out—yet we now see that at least one side of the equation cannot be measured reliably. One of the simple solutions is to stop trying to quantify exercise this way. Not only is caloric-expenditure measurement faulty, but it also fails to take into account the exercise-induced increase in metabolic rate or the fact that when you build muscle, you burn more energy at rest. So if you must have a metric to chase, make sure calories isn't it.

When Andy was training for the 2007 national weightlifting championships, he needed to lose weight in the run-up to the competition to be eligible in the sixty-nine-kilogram division. As part of this effort, he started recording his weight every day at the same time for a month. Andy found that his weight went down by 0.2–0.3 pounds every day Monday through Friday, and then increased by 0.3–0.4 pounds on Saturday and Sunday. However, when he compared his weight on the first Monday to the second, third, and fourth Mondays, he noticed that his weight loss occurred almost as a weekly drop, despite the day-to-day and weekend variations. This shows that weight loss is not always linear. Someone who didn't understand this (as Andy did) might have incorrectly assumed that their program wasn't working and that they needed to change it.

During this time, Andy wasn't counting calories but rather just paying attention to how he felt each day. If he felt like

Follow the Fashion

Fitness companies have always wanted celebrity endorsers to hawk their wares, knowing that when people see their favorite athletes or celebrities promoting a certain product, they're going to want it too. The same goes for wearables, which have become the latest fashion accessory that we just cannot live without. Recognizing that putting an ugly piece of plastic on your wrist is just about the opposite of New York Fashion Week chic, technology makers have signed up big-name designers to come up with bejeweled and bedazzled versions that one company claims will take you from "run to runway."

Certain smartphones and smartwatches were already status symbols to some. With wearables now getting in the act, it seems that being active isn't enough—you have to look good doing it and let people know that you're getting fit fashionably. Putting a wearable on your wrist has become a social signifier that (we hope) tells the world, "I'm fit and active!" There's nothing wrong with a well-designed, good-looking product (see the iPhone), but such a marketing ploy is just adding to our obsession with image. If you want to put something on your wrist that looks expensive and signals to others how successful you are, you've got plenty of options at your local jewelry store. If you'd rather focus on your health, ditch the fashion accessories altogether and get moving!

crap during or after a hard workout, he remedied this by eating more. If he stopped losing weight, he ate a little less. The emphasis was on daily self-assessment of his overall well-being, not on calories in and out, yet he achieved his goal. When you consider that we naturally overestimate how many calories we burn during exercise and often combine this delusion with the exaggeration that fitness trackers and exercise equipment provide (cardio machines overestimated caloric burn by an average of 19 percent, according to one study conducted at UC San Francisco's Human Performance Center), I think Andy pursued a better, more conscious path to his goal.[20]

Misguided Guidelines

As helpful as it may seem to have a device monitor how close you are to certain health goals, it's important to consider whether those goals are really what you should be aiming for. Are they based on data? Do they apply to you personally, not just the average person? And if so, do you possess the knowledge to interpret the data and apply it to your training?

Ten Thousand Steps and the New RDAs of Fitness

In 1927, Lawrence Henderson, David Dill, John Talbott, and Arlie Bock decided they needed to study the limits of the human body in more depth, and so they founded the Harvard Fatigue Laboratory (HFL). This is arguably the birthplace of the modern study of physiology, but while sports performance is one of the biggest focuses of equivalent modern labs, Henderson and company were more concerned with the impact of bodily limitations on output and recovery in industry and combat. Rather than trying to find the minimum effective dose of activity, nutrition, temperature stimulation, and so on, the scientists at the HFL wanted their test subjects to go to extremes to see what was possible and how far you could push body and mind before one or both broke.[21]

If the HFL were still around, there's no way its overseers would get away with replicating those studies from the mid-

1900s, because they'd be condemned as dangerous. The scientists' "hot room" regularly subjected study participants to temperatures up to 115 degrees while the cold chamber chilled them to −40 degrees. To make sure their conclusions weren't just theoretical, the HFL team replicated them in nature. They took subjects to Newfoundland to see how long they could endure being immersed in snow, so they could give the US military guidelines on winter clothing, and led them up peaks in New Hampshire's White Mountains to see what amount of insulation was needed for army boots. They also came up with new formulas for survival rations by depriving people of food for days or feeding them only pemmican, a high-fat and protein-rich dried subsistence food used by the Inuit during long expeditions (like the elven lembas bread the hobbits used in *The Lord of the Rings,* if it was a mixture of powdered dried meat and animal fat).[22]

Out of the HFL's studies in the extreme came recommendations for everyday life. The most famous of these is the Recommended Dietary Allowance (RDA) of micronutrients, still found on food and supplement labels today. These numbers were set at the minimum intake needed to prevent disease. So the vitamin C baseline of sixty milligrams per day is the least you should consume to stop yourself from getting scurvy.

In the past few years, the fitness industry has come up with something similar for movement: activity-based RDAs that aim to get us back up to the basal metabolic rates that we used to have back when we had more physically challenging jobs and lifestyles. Chief among these are the prescriptions for ten thousand steps a day and thirty minutes of daily exercise, which have, through years of repetition, become pervasive, readily accepted, and rarely questioned.

When it comes to nutrient RDAs, very few people obsessively read labels and add together foods to total 100 percent of the recommended amounts of vitamins C and A, iron, or the rest. Instead, we know that we need these micronutrients and so try to eat a balanced, healthy diet. A similar mind-set should apply to activity-focused RDAs. While some might find the ten-thousand-steps and thirty-minutes rules helpful at first, they should aim to replace these rudimentary guidelines with a lifestyle that includes plenty of untracked daily activity. Anything prescribed as a society-wide guideline is conceived to influence a majority of people positively, using bare minimums. This can be very useful on a policy level, but such recommendations should not be misinterpreted as a blueprint for performance progress or excellence. Instead, they're just a baseline requirement for the average person. And you don't want to settle for average, do you?

Furthermore, if you're going to use wearable technology to measure something, it shouldn't be the number of steps you take (once you have a rough sense of what level of movement such a total requires). Accumulating ten thousand steps a day might help sedentary people lose weight initially, if combined with a better diet and other kinds of physical exertion, but such early progress will quickly level off and they'll need more resistance training and intense interval work to overcome stagnation.

220 Minus Age: The Max Heart Rate Mistake

One of the most misleading and yet longest-standing health myths is that the fastest pulse your heart is capable of reaching is found by a simple equation: 220 minus your age. This calculation has its roots in the work of Indiana University exercise physiologist and former Olympic runner Sid Robinson in the 1930s.[23] But it wasn't until a later review of data compiled in 1971 and the subsequent creation of "a line of best fit"—a straight line that represents the overall data on a graph with many points—that the equation was made public and became an accepted standard among coaches in all sports.

The problem is that the numbers collected in these studies were almost all based on observational studies rather than actual heart rate testing of various age groups and the statistics that such scientific work would've provided.[24] And yet, like any myth, once it became accepted by the coaching fraternity and drilled into their athletes for the next forty-five years, the 220-minus-age falsehood became extremely difficult to counter, even for those who collected evidence that contradicted it. As a result, we've had several generations whose training has been limited by this glass ceiling of what their coaches thought was their cardiac threshold. Just like one-rep max lifts in a weight room, the 220-minus-age number was considered 100 percent effort, and heart-rate zone programs worked backwards as percentages of this.

But if, say, a twenty-year-old athlete was actually able to raise and maintain their heart rate beyond the 200 "max" that the formula presented, then even their high-intensity sessions would have fallen short of the stimuli needed to produce the best possible physiological adaptations—effectively leaving some degree of untapped performance potential on the table. I know firsthand how faulty the equation is from spending time with Don Wildman, the founder of the fitness chain that's now Bally's. At age eighty-two, Don snowboards more than eighty days a year and surfs, bikes, and runs on many more. Surging ahead of athletes half his age, Don's heart rate goes and stays way above the 130-something that his max is supposed to be. And he's not some freakish outlier, either. A study Andy published recently found that the average max heart rate for eighty-one-year-old lifelong athletes was 160 beats per minute, 21 above the 220-minus-age estimate (it's worth noting that even nonathletes in this study topped out at 146 beats per minute, which is still higher than that calculation).[25]

This inaccuracy of the 220-minus-age equation pertains to the heart rate monitoring features still used in today's latest technology. If their algorithms are based on this faulty formula, then the advice—"Go faster!" or "Slow down!"—that they're pumping into our headphones (or devices the cool kids are calling "hearables") is based on a faulty premise. As are the ranges for heart rate zone training. Until now we've regarded the accuracy of our wearables with an unquestioning attitude, blindly believing that they're inerrant. But we know for a fact that the max heart rate calculation is faulty, and it's only a matter of time before we realize that some of the other exercise formulas we've accepted as truth all these years are also way off. This means that the devices we've come to rely on to guide us might not be leading us to better health and performance but rather up the garden path.

If you're determined to utilize your max heart rate in your training, don't rely on the 220-minus-age equation. Instead, just do an all-out interval workout and record your upper limit, and then have an experienced coach write you a program that works backwards from this to set more realistic and beneficial training zones.

Listen to Your Heart (and Your Other Instincts)

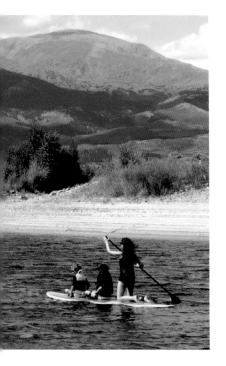

Since Seppo Säynäjäkangas introduced the first wireless heart rate monitor in 1977, coaches have been convinced that basing their athletes' training on specific, measurable outputs will yield better performance outcomes. Thus came the popularity of focusing endurance athletes' work on heart-rate zones, which in turn spawned efforts to train different metabolic systems depending on the sport of choice and individual competitors' strengths and weaknesses.

Almost forty years after Säynäjäkangas's invention birthed chest straps, wrist-worn monitors, and, most recently, smartphone and smartwatch apps, we're starting to realize how limited heart rate–based training actually is, and how much time and potential we've wasted in fixating on it. As far back as 1992, scientific studies began showing that when athletes train based on how hard they feel a session is—what we refer to as rate of perceived effort (RPE)—it's just as effective as trying to keep their heart rate in a certain zone for a predetermined length of time.

Such research demonstrates that we have significantly underestimated how capable our bodies are of perceiving the stimuli we're subjected to and how this can inform what we do, how often we do it, and the amount of effort we exert on any given day. It comes down to a battle between measuring and feeling. Many so-called experts in exercise science and the fitness industry would like us to believe that we can only progress and adapt if our training is based on biomarkers and data. Yet clinical trials prove that this is not the case.[26]

The trouble is that many athletes have spent years or even decades mired in measurables and so have unwittingly dulled their awareness of what their body is trying to tell them. Our innate ability to assess how we're moving through space never diminishes, but our capacity to pay attention to the resulting feedback and act accordingly certainly does. We think that the machines exist to serve us, but when it comes to gauging how activity feels as part of a holistic experience, we've started serving the machines. That's why we need to get back in touch with our natural awareness and instincts, instead of always deferring to the electronic second brain wrapped around our wrists. So if you do collect your heart-rate information, review it after your workout, not while you should be focusing on your own movement and your environment during the session.

Messing with Your Mind

For five years, I collected daily heart-rate data on myself and the athletes I was coaching, believing that obsessively detailing this measurable would enable me to tailor our training. But one day I had an epiphany, and just like that, me and heart rate monitoring were through. A friend of mine wanted to start doing triathlons and asked me to go running with him. I readily agreed, and we set off for a ten-mile loop around Newport Beach's Back Bay. He asked me to slow down and I did for a while, then gradually increased the pace again when I thought he was ready for it. Yet soon enough, he piped up again, "I've gotta go slower." I repeated the slow-down, speed-up cycle, and he finally started freaking out as he frantically looked at his wearable every few seconds. "Brian, if we don't back off the pace I'm going to blow up," he said desperately. "My heart rate is in the 160s!"

I thought about it for a second and then told him, "If you were about to blow up, we wouldn't be having this conversation." Once you reach a certain metabolic limit, you're not able to utter more than a couple of words, and even that would be difficult. Yet here we were, having a back-and-forth conversation, without him gasping for breath or straining to get his words out. Simply put, the monitor was misleading him into thinking that he was maxed out, when in fact he was far fitter than he or the device was giving him credit for.

From that day on, I stopped using heart rate to measure intensity. It is one possible measurement for this, but, as the unnecessary midrun panic showed, not an entirely accurate one. I've found that looking at power output (often displayed as watts on a rowing machine or Assault AirBike if you're indoors, or numerous tracking devices if you're outdoors) and rpm for cycling is a much better gauge of intensity. Periodically I break out a heart rate monitor to see if where I'm at metabolically correlates with my beats per minute.

And then I find that a funny thing happens. Just as my friend did on that run, I start freaking out if my heart rate gets in the 160s, believing that I'm approaching my body's limit. But then my rational brain kicks in and tells me that this instinct is wrong because I'm usually not near my max power output or speed. This shows how the mind can use technology to start playing tricks on you, which in turn enables you to make excuses about why you need to stop or dial back your intensity. Try experimenting with your own power output without a heart rate monitor, and then look at your bpm to see if a similar thing happens to you and if there's a disconnect between what the display tells you and what you know you're capable of. You can also utilize the talk test to see how hard you're going. If you're chattering away as my friend was in the example above, you're only at a low to moderate level of intensity. If it's difficult to say anything, you're likely above 80 percent effort.

Torturing the Data

Data inaccuracy is but one of the many potential problems with using a metrics-driven approach to fitness. There's also the potential issue of manipulating the numbers. Tim Ferriss explains: "I don't like to gather tons of numbers and then look for meaning in the numbers, because you can torture the data to find just about anything you want to find. Maybe you have a confirmation bias and want to find something in the data. You can bend it and manipulate it, and slice and dice it in such a way, or just fool yourself in such a fashion that you'll find patterns and create cause and effect where there is none."[27]

The solution? Cultivating both intellectual honesty and a controlled approach to self-experimentation. Ferriss continues, "Richard Feynman said, 'The first principle is that you must not fool yourself—and you are the easiest person to fool.' Good scientific method helps protect you against this. You've also got to develop your thought processes in such a way so that you don't fool yourself. It also helps me to focus on a specific objective. All the metrics I gather and the testing I do—let's say a biopsy is looking at citrate synthase or VO_2 max—is goal-oriented."[28]

If you are going to do any kind of performance-based test, make sure you have a defined purpose, objective, and hypothesis before testing. Then, have a clear action plan that you are willing to commit to afterward, regardless of the outcome. If you can't do this, you're acknowledging your confirmation bias and that you were only looking to hear what you wanted to hear, instead of going into the test with an open mind and searching for a real solution.

All too often when we test ourselves or, as coaches, test our athletes, we're trying to find something that is obvious even without any kind of test. For example, Andy does a lot of work with fighters. One of them was trying to come back from elbow surgery that'd led to a long training layoff. He was out of shape and fifty pounds overweight and asked Andy to test his VO_2 max. Andy refused. Why? Because he knew the fighter's injury history and how it had disrupted his preparation and, just using his eyes, could tell that he was too heavy and unfit.

However, he did run this test on a few other fighters because even though they were in great shape, he started noticing some performance issues with their conditioning that couldn't be pinpointed with simple observation alone. The VO_2 max test helped identify their issue, and the fighters' coaches spent the next six weeks acting on this insight with a specific plan, after which the problems went away. Andy had a hunch that came from watching the athlete through the lens of many years' experience, and the test confirmed it—not the other way around. The lesson is that you should use technology to see what your eyes can't, but recognize that it's still only a tool to find data that a coach must then use to inform your programming.

The Limits of Scientific Studies

Objective data from scientific studies is essential for any area of research, whether it's the effects of a certain nutritional supplement or how subatomic particles behave. But when it comes to health and fitness, marketing and media hyperbole can lead to misunderstandings and misguided action. We may think we're doing something great for our bodies, but are we treating symptoms instead of the cause, or even interfering in a natural and positive bodily process? Is a product promising the world without delivering? A healthy skepticism and willingness to experiment can help separate the scientific wheat from the chaff.

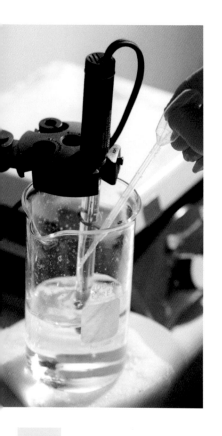

Doing the Dishes with a Hammer

Imagine you're asked by a company that makes tools to see if their new hammer "works." You could go one of two ways when looking into the usefulness of the hammer. First, you could pound nails into planks of wood. "Yep," you'd tell the company's owners, "this hammer works for pounding nails." But what if instead you focused your efforts on trying to wash the dirty dishes in your kitchen sink with that same hammer? You'd come back with a report stating that the tool was useless.

This analogy might seem a little silly, but it applies quite well to the field of exercise science. Every fitness wearable or supplement "works" in some way or another. It's just a question of whether this functionality lines up with how the company is marketing its products and the path chosen by the research scientists who looked into its effectiveness.

So if Andy were going to study the benefits of tart cherry juice, he wouldn't investigate potential benefits that he knows aren't going to materialize, such as increased protein synthesis. Instead, he'd look at the existing literature and home in on a likely use for tart cherry extract, like reducing inflammation. Then he would set up a study with two groups, one that would take a certain dose of the extract after exercising and one that wouldn't. He'd likely find that tart cherry does indeed reduce inflammation biomarkers.[29]

You should be very cautious of clickbait titles, sensationalized news headlines, and anything heralding the discovery of a new miracle cure. Instead, it'd be better to become your own experiment (à la Tim Ferriss in *The 4-Hour Body*) and approach all potential solutions to a specific issue (like inflammation, poor sleep, or lethargy) with healthy skepticism. Many technologies help fix a single issue at best, and many more merely cover up symptoms without resolving the root of the problem.

Efficacy and Elixirs of Life

The trouble comes when we try to extrapolate the efficacy that science supports. So if Andy publishes his study showing that tart cherry juice reduces inflammation and the company making the extract, which funded the research, incorporates this into the marketing for their new product, that's fine. But if they use Andy's work to try to justify the claim that tart cherry extract reverses the effects of aging and can make you look ten years younger after just two weeks, they've gone too far.

Unfortunately, this is often what happens with wearables, supplements, and other products promoted within the fitness industry and on the mass market. Their makers effectively become the same kind of snake oil salesmen who promised cure-alls to people in the eighteenth, nineteenth, and early twentieth centuries. Until a class action lawsuit pops up in the news, there's little restriction on such wild claims, as long as the manufacturer is careful to attach the relevant disclaimer (such as "These statements have not been evaluated by the Food and Drug Administration") on the label.

It's the responsibility of manufacturers to stay within the boundaries of reality with how they market and label products, but it's up to you as the consumer to set your BS filter to "high" and question what appear to be sensationalist claims. If a product's promises seem too good to be true, they likely are. If you want to fact-check the maker's claims, skip the scientific journal articles that read like they've been written in Klingon. Rather, try to find a blog post or podcast that features the scientist whose research supposedly proves the efficacy of the product you're curious about. See what they have to say about its usefulness and limitations, and then make up your own mind. Also remember that any supplement—whether it's tart cherry extract or anything else—should be a short-term fix for a specific problem. If you stop taking it after a while and the symptoms—inflammation or poor sleep, for example—return, then you haven't addressed the real issue and need to try changing your lifestyle or training habits.

Another way that we misinterpret scientific studies and the resulting media hyperbole is that all too often we fundamentally misunderstand how our bodies function. For example, many people don't realize that the inflammatory response is critical to survival and progress. It's the only way that your body knows how to adapt to a training stimulus. So if you deploy technology that focuses on reducing or delaying your natural inflammation response, you'll never truly progress.

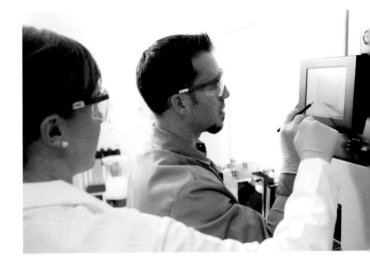

The research on muscle hypertrophy (growth) shows this quite clearly, and we now know that taking supplements that have some anti-inflammatory benefits, like resveratrol, can actually shift our muscle fiber profile.[30] Simply put, even technologies that work wonders in certain ways can have disadvantages or unintended consequences. Because we don't fully understand these yet, you should embrace any new technology slowly and not look at it as a magic bullet.

One piece of technology that can help you improve your understanding (and fine-tune your BS filter) is the internet. Websites like www.examine.com use teams of scientists and PhDs to provide a layman's synopsis of each study and its findings. Other sites, like www.researchgate.net, provide access to the full research article if you want to read more. In addition, sites like Dr. Chris Beardsley and Dr. Bret Contreras's www.strengthandconditioningresearch.com and Dr. Yann Le Meur's www.ylmsportscience.com (and their corresponding social media feeds) have started making highly informative and yet easy-to-understand infographics for studies on sport science, nutrition, health, and the human body. The pioneer in this area is Alan Aragon, who has been interpreting research for the masses for years on his popular blog, www.alanaragon.com.

We Can't Wait for Tomorrow to Arrive

Though the gulf between scientific research and practical application is closing, coaches and athletes can't wait for science to give a definitive answer before we act. Otherwise we'd have to tell everyone, "We're not certain what's best, so just sit on your couch until we figure it out." No! We've all got to get out and move more and rely on technology less. In doing so, we recognize that yes, we'll definitely make some mistakes. But we'll learn as much if not more from these as we will from our successes, and so we'll make progress long before science confirms what we find to be self-evident. The key is to put on your shoes, get out the door, and begin. Keep your ears and eyes open so you're able to absorb new information, but make sure that your quest for new information doesn't produce inertia.

Be Your Own Experiment

As the wearables revolution has taken hold, we've become too beholden to our technology. In doing so, we've abdicated our power and freely given away responsibility for our health. To reclaim yourself, you need to ask a very simple question about your physical practice: what works for *you*? (And of course its corollary: what doesn't?) It's time to take charge of your own learning again and begin figuring things out through exploration and discovery, rather than just relying on a digital coaching program to make all the decisions. This can be as simple or sophisticated as you want. Maybe it's as easy as tracking your mood, on a scale of one to ten, every morning. Or if you're a data guy or girl, perhaps you chart and plot everything—sleep, mood, body weight, exercise performance, resting heart rate, desire to train, and sense of fulfillment—on a spreadsheet. If such information gathering motivates you and helps you continually improve, there's no harm in it.

Cheat Mortality, Not Your Wallet

In recent years, testing companies have taken advantage of athletes' relentless pursuit of progress and come up with all sorts of fancy tests. If you want to fork over a few hundred bucks and get back a nice, fancy spreadsheet full of graphs and charts, far be it from labs to deny you the pleasure. And yet, despite the broad range of measurements now available and the eye-catching ways of presenting them, the four best predictors of mortality are unchanged from fifty years ago. They're still:

- VO_2 max
- leg strength
- lean body mass
- grip strength

Instead of wasting your hard-earned cash on a battery of exhaustive (and, often, exhausting) tests, you can get almost any lab to perform the four listed above for less than fifty dollars and in just fifteen to twenty minutes. If you find that you're lacking in any or all of these areas, get with a strength and conditioning coach and ask him or her to devise a program that syncs up progress in them with your other health and performance goals.

You can also do basic versions of these four tests yourself. For VO_2 max, use the four-hundred-meter walk test and six-minute walk/run test, or the two-thousand-meter time trial on a rowing machine, from which Concept2's calculator will estimate your VO_2 max, at http://www.concept2.com/indoor-rowers/training/calculators/vo2max-calculator.[31] A low-cost option to measure your grip strength is a handheld dynamometer, which will only cost you twenty-five to fifty dollars. At the other end of the scale, if you're a pro athlete who wants deeper understanding of your physiology, you could go to most exercise physiology labs and get a battery of tests done, including an ultrasound or MRI to measure muscle mass, DEXA for total lean body mass, and a metabolic cart for

VO_2 max. In addition, you could get your strength tested on an isokinetic dynamometer or, better yet, a force plate with motion capture to assess movement technique/quality. Such a range of tests will usually cost between $1,500 and $2,000.

Bragging Rights

If you spend any time on cycling, running, or triathlon forums online, you'll see many multipage threads on VO_2 max numbers. While this can be a valid test if you use it to learn about your limits and then train to push them, for many, a high score is just something to brag about. I've seen firsthand that a lot of people who get tested and try to put the number to use in lactate threshold–based training never retest to see how they've changed their bodies. So they cling to this old number for months or years and waste hours and hours of training time on trying to move forward from a point that they've long since surpassed. As with any other physical test, obtaining a VO_2 max score should be a learning opportunity. If you're going to do it and then "train to the test," you should get retested every three to four weeks to see what your new capacity is and then adjust your training strategy accordingly. And while you're at it, skip the self-aggrandizing forum posts!

Greed Is the Game

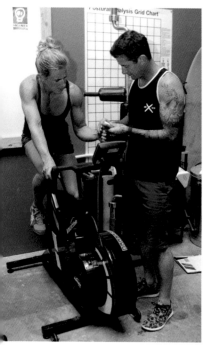

In addition to calling our self-awareness into question, the wearables revolution also presents ethical issues regarding the privacy, security, and availability of performance and health-related data. Does a company that makes fitness wearables have the right to mix your data with those of other users to improve its software or conduct research, or even the right to sell the information to a third party? You don't have to be a modern George Orwell to have serious concerns about the answer to such questions, which, to date, manufacturers of fitness tech have failed to address. NBA players seem to share these worries: their December 2016 collective bargaining agreement included the formation of a wearables committee to oversee the use of devices and the data they harvest.[32]

If one of the most popular and powerful sports leagues in the world is having trouble getting to grips with the privacy issues that self-quantification presents, what about the rest of us who don't have the power of renowned athletes to demand change? What happens to all that information about you and me that our devices are collecting around the clock? Well, it doesn't just disappear. The companies who make your favorite gizmos are storing every byte on a server somewhere. What happens next is anyone's guess.

On the positive side, such organizations are using information about your body and its performance to improve the algorithms that provide you with real-time advice on what to do and how to do it. But is that all that's happening with this most personal of information? According to an extensive December 2016 study by the Center for Digital Democracy, they're also looking to profit from your data. The report states that wearables "are already being integrated into a growing Big Data digital health and marketing ecosystem, which is focused on gathering and *monetizing personal and health data* in order to influence consumer behavior" [emphasis added].[33] So soon you'll be receiving ads sold to the highest bidders and delivered right to your wrist. These will be based on your health issues, the activities you partake in, and your location and could cover everything from drugs to more technology to fitness clothing and gear, and who knows what else.

The study's authors also predict that as wearables become more sophisticated, the number of threats to your privacy will increase and diversify: "Biosensors will routinely be able to capture not only an individual's heart rate, body temperature, and movement, but also brain activity, moods, and emotions. These data can, in turn, be combined with personal information from other sources—including health-care providers and drug companies—raising such potential harms as discriminatory profiling, manipulative marketing, and security breaches."[34]

When you purchased your fitness tracker, you likely thought it would improve your health and give you some motivation to move more and eat better. That might be true to some extent, but if this report and others like it are correct, technology companies are using such promises as a Trojan horse. Once it's attached to your wrist, the true goal becomes clear: get as much of your data as possible, package it, and sell it for whatever the going rate is. Without so much as pausing to ask you if you're okay with that—which I'm certainly not.

As the authors of the Center for Digital Democracy report insist, either these organizations need to agree to a code of ethics voluntarily and be monitored by an independent third party, or the government needs to step in with sweeping legislation. This would require the makers of fitness-tracking devices to stop selling consumer information and to start sharing openly what exactly they're planning to do with your data. There also need to be strict and enforceable restrictions on advertising and marketing, with safeguards in place to make sure companies aren't discriminating based on your demographics. If we want to protect our children, we must also demand that ads delivered to wearables are not targeting kids.

Where Do I Sign?

When you go to a doctor's office or hospital, many of the forms you fill out concern the privacy of your health data and your permission to let that provider use it. In addition to filling out a HIPAA (Health Insurance Portability and Accountability Act) form every year, you also give your consent for whatever procedure or test you're going to have done that day. There are many flaws in our health-care system, but at least there's some regulatory oversight and mandatory procedures regarding data sharing, privacy, and protection.

Not so in the world of fitness technology. While you imply that you're giving a company permission to monitor you and collect your biometrics just by purchasing their devices, you never have the chance to sign any kind of permission form or waiver. So they're gathering information on your biology around the clock for as long as you use their products. If wearables for kids take off—and the brightly colored, "fun" designs now being introduced implies that they will—your children could conceivably submit to an entire lifetime's worth of monitoring. Surely this should require the signature of a parent or guardian on some kind of consent form, just like when you take your kids to the doctor's office? The same goes for your data and mine. Swiping your credit card to purchase a wearable or phone app should not give companies free rein to collect, distribute, and profit from your health data. And yet for the time being, this is the only assent you're giving them to do just that.

I Want It All, and I Want It Now

All but three states in the US have laws on their books concerning citizens' access to their medical information that either meet or exceed the HIPAA nationwide standard for electronic medical record (EMR) access, which stipulates that you have "the right to inspect, review, and receive a copy of your medical records and billing records that are held by health plans and health care providers covered by the Privacy Rule," according to the US Department of Health and Human Services.[35] If you ask a hospital for your records, they have to provide them in their entirety. Several states stipulate a fifteen-day limit for doing so, others thirty days, and some a "reasonable time frame." While this isn't the kind of instant access we might want, at least the information is available and there are regulatory consequences should a health-care practitioner fail to provide it.[36]

This isn't the case for fitness tracking. The poet Ted Hughes said, "I hope each of us owns the facts of his or her life." But when it comes to the information collected by wearables and apps, it's unclear who owns the facts, or even has access to them.[37] At the time of writing, there was no federal or state legislation covering requests for information or the delivery of this data. These organizations might claim that they already share your data with you, but showing you daily, weekly, and monthly snapshots in charts and graphs is hardly full disclosure; these likely represent less than 1 percent of the total information collected. There needs to be some government oversight here. It seems reasonable to give fitness tracking companies a thirty-day limit to send you all your data in a standardized format once you've requested it. After all, you never gave them permission to gather it in the first place, and while they're storing the information, it is *your* data, not theirs.

Under Lock and Key

Another disturbing element of data collection is the security of that information, or lack thereof. We'd like to assume that fitness technology companies are using the latest encryption, bulletproof firewalls, and airtight, backed-up servers, but this could very well be wishful thinking. The reality is that we have no idea how safe or unsafe our health information is once it's sent off into the digital ether. When a hospital has a data breach or someone hacks into your credit card provider's database, it's a big deal that often comes with hefty fines. Have wearables and app manufacturers been the victims of similar cyberattacks, and if so, what are they now doing differently to prevent further breaches? We just don't know because the media isn't reporting this kind of news. There should be federal and state standards for this kind of health data, as there are for medical and financial information, and in addition, the press needs to do a better job of investigating such issues. This isn't a call for muckraking journalism or whistle-blowers to share secrets, but rather for our Fourth Estate to do a better job of keeping its readers informed.

Demanding Disclosure

While the policy wonks in our nation's capital can probably come up with enough regulations to fill a phone book, I think every manufacturer of fitness technology owes it to their customers to make a simple pledge: "We promise to make all the data we collect public." You're doing them the favor of paying a couple of hundred bucks for a device that probably costs twenty dollars to make, and throwing your very heart (rate) into the bargain. In return, they offer some very generic guidance while collecting and putting to use very detailed data.

It's time to make this a better deal for us, the consumers. Opening up the data vaults would not only fulfill what I believe is an ethical obligation to openness and transparency but also enable people to study the information and use it to improve health care, public wellness, and sports performance. Researchers would no longer have to make the effort to put together small test and control groups who participate in limited, short-term studies, because they'd be able to run the numbers on millions of people's biometrics over many years. This would lead to many breakthroughs that might otherwise have taken years to achieve. If these companies are really trying to help us, let them prove it.

Wearables at Work

It's not just the use of wearables in people's private lives that faces scrutiny. An increasing number of companies are encouraging their employees to use a device at work and outside it as part of their corporate wellness initiatives. This is a big win for fitness device manufacturers, one of which specifically outlined such company plans as one of their five main goals when they went public.[38] An additional bonus is that large organizations gather data from their employees' devices around the clock, information that fitness technology peddlers aggregate and feed into their ever-growing data pools.

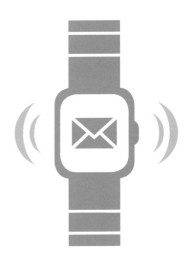

The main benefit for companies whose staff don wearables is that monitoring employee health enables them to score discounts from health insurance providers; they're also able to write off the devices as a business expense. However, some companies are using wearables to track the location of their employees in an effort to increase productivity. One example is Amazon, whose thousands of warehouse employees wear GPS tags integrated with a handheld scanner that provides them with the fastest path to the next item they need to pull from the shelves.[39]

Such a use seems perfectly reasonable, as does utilizing navigational aids for delivery services; safety devices for miners, oil rig staff, soldiers, and others who work in hazardous environments; and wearable cameras for emergency services personnel (although the latter continues to be controversial). But what about the use of fitness trackers for regular office workers?

The Guardian shared a story of one London analytics company that required its employees to participate in a self-quantification project. The founder told the reporter that if anyone "didn't want to do it, they were out."[40] Can a company legally terminate an employee who doesn't want to use a wearable? This seems like a lawsuit waiting to happen.

Compulsory participation is just the tip of the ethical iceberg. Should an employer have the right to collect their employees' biometrics, and if so, how should they be allowed to use this information? How can they ensure that personal health data isn't used in a prejudicial or discriminatory fashion (like at one data science company, which used such information to tag employees with labels like "Busy and Coping" and "Irritated and Unsettled")?[41] Is it okay for them to share the data with third parties, whether for analysis or any other purpose? What security measures do they have in place to protect the privacy of their employees? To date, few organizations or regulatory entities seem willing to consider, let alone answer, any of these pressing questions.

Someone who did is *Financial Times* journalist Sarah O'Connor. She spent a week tethered to multiple wearables and after seven days submitted the data to her editor. During the experiment, she continually updated a Facebook page, did interviews with other media outlets, and posted a series of stories on the topic. In a podcast for NPR, O'Connor said, "It felt very weird, and actually, I really didn't like the feeling at all. It just felt as if my job was suddenly leaking into every area of my life. Like on the Thursday night, a good friend and colleague had a 30th birthday party, and I went along. And it got to sort of 1 o'clock, and I realized I was panicking about my sleep monitor and what it was going to look like the next day."[42]

While some of her younger colleagues thought the experiment was a good thing, O'Connor relayed the consensus among newsroom veterans that self-monitoring was an "awful infringement of your civil liberties and your privacy and your dignity." One coworker issued a damning indictment of wearables in the workplace in general: "The employment relationship is like this—I give you the work, and you give me the money. Anything else and you can go to hell."[43]

O'Connor chose to discontinue her personal wearables experiment once the week was over. Yet the larger, society-wide study still continues apace, as more and more companies make fitness technology part of their wellness plans. While I disagree with the premise of collecting employees' health data, my disapproval isn't going to make it go away. On a more practical level, any company that's considering the use of fitness technology should make it voluntary. Every employee who wishes to participate should be given a consent form that clearly explains the type of information that will be collected, who will be able to view it, and what it will be used for. The company should also pledge to keep the data secure, to not share it with any third parties, and to not use it as part of performance evaluations. Such statements might not stand up in court, but they would at least offer employees some level of assurance that the company has good intentions.

Blue Is the Color

The sky is blue, the sea is blue, your eyes might be blue. Or so you think. One of the most interesting podcasts I've listened to in ages was a *Radiolab* episode about colors. The presenters shared the revelation that for a long time, humans didn't call the color blue by name. In fact, ancient texts—including Homer's *The Odyssey*—make no reference to it. Homer referred to the sea as "wine-dark" and the sky as white. And it's not just the ancient world that didn't include *blue* in their color vocabulary; the lexicon of some African tribes still omits it. I'm not making this up—listen to the podcast![44]

It wasn't until merchants in the Far and Middle East started dyeing clothes blue that we started paying attention to it. Part of the reason is that the kind of bright, unfiltered blues we put in clothing, on book covers, and in so many other places don't occur that often in nature. Contrast this to red, which is nature's danger signal in some poisonous berries, venomous animals, and such, which we had to pay more attention to and name early in our species' development of language for self-preservation purposes. Once Gutenberg's printing press became popular and the Bible—which mentions blue—went global, we finally had a widely distributed text that referenced blue as a distinct color. Soon after, other books followed suit, and blue and its derivatives (who doesn't love Majorelle blue?) entered everyday language.

The fact that it took people thousands of years to notice and name the different shades of blue indicates that we're missing a lot of other things in the world around us. For our purposes in this book, if you unplug from your fitness tracker when you go outside and start looking and listening more intently, you'll pick up on small things with your eyes and ears that you would never have seen had you been connected to technology. The more you pay attention to what your body is perceiving in the world around you, the more sensitive you will become. As naturalist Dick Proenneke said, "Nature provides so many things, if one has the eye to notice them."

Perhaps as you're unplugged in nature you'll notice when you're hyperventilating, which burns extra energy, or recognize when your gait or paddling technique is falling apart. Does this really mean you need a day off, or are you just sleepy, dehydrated, or undernourished? Look at your sleep, drinking, and eating patterns and make your own judgment.

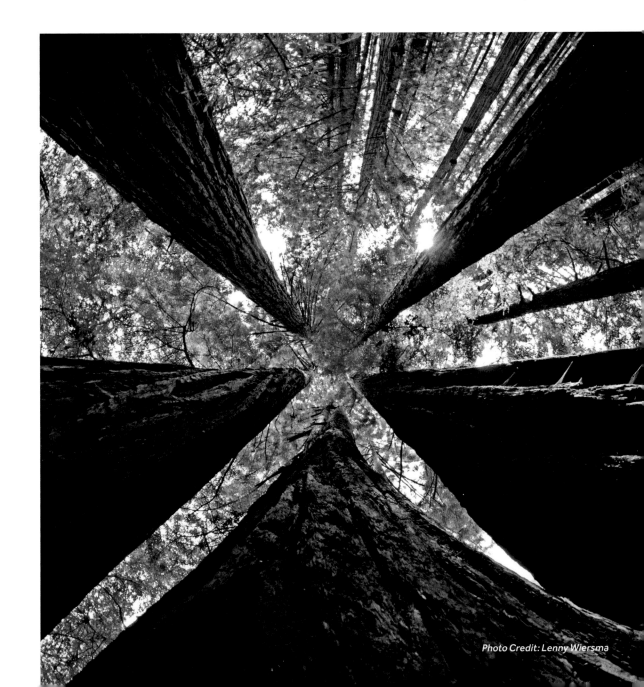

Photo Credit: Lenny Wiersma

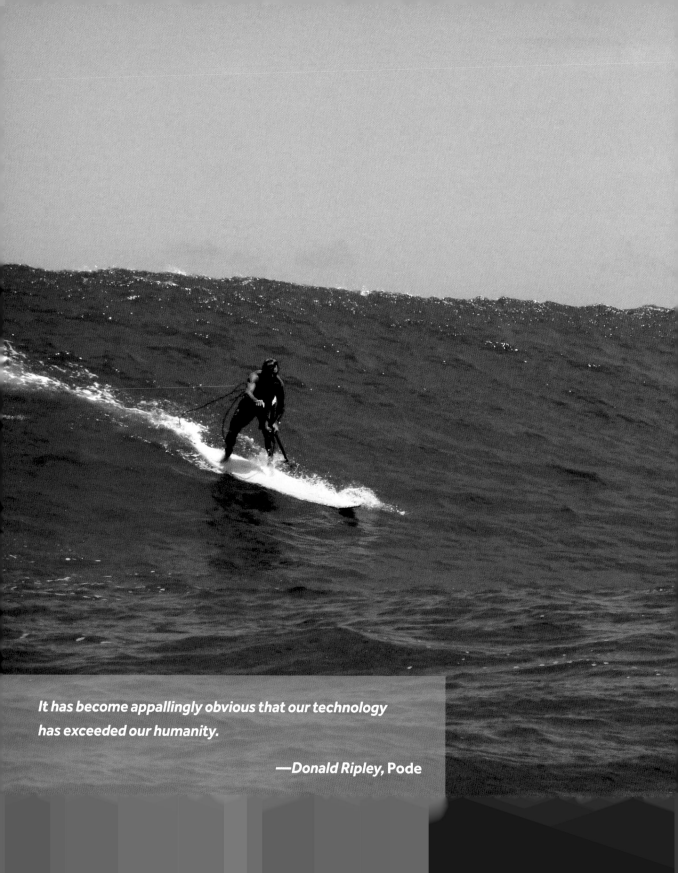

It has become appallingly obvious that our technology has exceeded our humanity.

—**Donald Ripley, Pode**

CHAPTER 2
REBOOTING YOUR TECH-ADDICTED PSYCHE

In her excellent book *Deep Nutrition,* Dr. Cate Shanahan states, "The age of technological health solutions has come to an end."[45] She goes on to explain that ever since the advances in medicine that followed World War II, we've increasingly placed more and more faith in the ability of technology to heal what ails us, and we've also given up personal responsibility for our health in favor of trusting the companies and government entities that provide these technologies and pharmaceuticals. And yet, despite the promise of progression, we're "sicker than ever."[46]

We're seeing a similar trend in the consumer electronics industry. We've elevated the CEOs of prominent tech companies to rock star status and hang on their every word. Their products permeate our every waking moment (and, in the case of sleep trackers, even our non-waking ones). While there are many ways that we can use technology positively, it can quickly also become a negative part of our lives. Before we know it, we're not just chasing more likes, shares, and retweets, reading and sending dozens of texts a day, and checking our e-mail because it's fun, but because we've become hooked on the little hits of happy hormones we get every time we do so.

Then you add fitness trackers, apps, and supposedly smart watches into the mix, and we merely extend and reinforce our compulsive, numbers-obsessed habits. As Adam Alter rightly states in his book *Irresistible,* we soon trade the potential for deep learning, skill development, and intrinsic reward that our training offers for "a sort of automatic mindlessness," which former *Psychology Today* editor Katherine Schreiber says is "the goal of addiction."[47] Then we combine our preexisting social-media fixation with our newfound fitness technology dependence, and get addiction squared.

Let's take a look at how we got to this point and what you can do to acknowledge, confront, and overcome the fitness tech addiction you might well have developed without even knowing it.

Taking the "Social" Out of "Social Media"

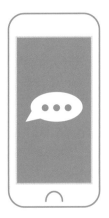

In the early days of the internet, its promise to bring us closer to each other, improve communication, and inspire new forms of community seemed boundless. These days, many of us know better. As wonderful as it is to be able to keep up with high school friends on Facebook or see what a celebrity had for lunch on Instagram, there's a darker side to social media.

Finding inspiration in the workout routine an actor or model posts on Twitter can quickly turn into an unhealthy fixation on aesthetics—can you get a six-pack like his or a butt like hers? Staying in touch with friends on Facebook can become an obsession with other people's lives and make it too easy to avoid authentic, face-to-face community. And our eagerness to share about our own lives can lead us to lose touch with the present moment and focus instead on how it's going to look on Instagram.

Narcissists Anonymous

It's no surprise that a study conducted by psychologists at Brunel University London found that narcissists were more likely to post about their fitness and diets to social media sites than those with less self-aggrandizing motivations. The report also found that narcissism was closely tied to low self-esteem.[48] Often, the data that fitness apps and wearables provide is just as misused as fuel for the workout-obsessed, body-fixated narcissists as the gym selfies they seem to never tire of posting. One of the Brunel researchers suggested that there's a simple fix to this issue: the narcissist's Facebook friends who are annoyed by the constant stream of look-at-me pictures should refuse to like or comment on them, and so stop enabling the poster's egotism.

Then there are the "famous for being famous" folks whose body-focused shots have gained millions of followers. If they were just posting photos of themselves, it would be easy enough to ignore them and move on. But it's the fact that many post fitness and nutrition tips to "get a body like mine"—or, in the lamentable case of the "belfie" posters, "a butt like mine"—that really bugs me. Their self-obsession and encouragement of others to imitate them reinforces our culture's fixation on aesthetics and how it is valued above real health.

Plus, the tips they provide are often way off the mark and frequently feature products they're paid to promote. While there's nothing wrong with looking good, this should be a by-product of a balanced and holistic lifestyle, not the be-all and end-all. But as long as we keep following these people (incidentally, even the term *following* sounds like stalking, doesn't it?) and asking for their advice, their influence will continue to increase and we'll end up even further from actual wellness and high performance.

This does *not* mean that just because some people have large social media followings and happen to look great, they are automatically devoid of useful information. In fact, several are very talented, intelligent, and highly successful coaches. The point we're making is that aesthetics should not be the criteria for how most people eat or train, as it provides the wrong target. It's absolutely fine for looks to be a strong motivation, but we have to realize the real goal is to improve our overall health and wellness. That way, if we fail to reach our aesthetic goal, we still end up happy because we have better energy, will live longer, and will perform better in whatever sport or activity we choose.

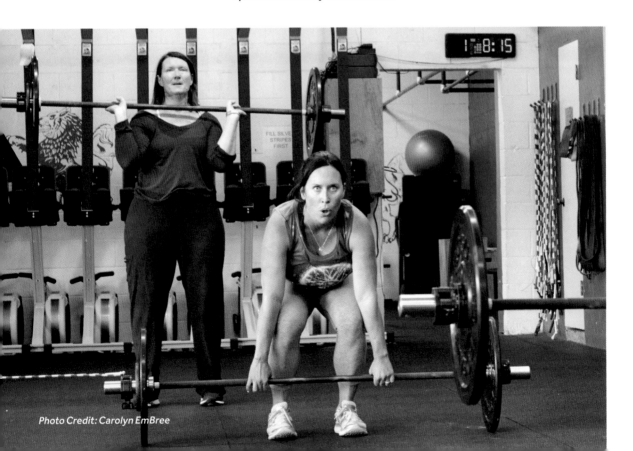

Photo Credit: Carolyn EmBree

One way to shift our focus from ourselves is to simply get out in what poet Robert Service calls "the Great Alone" and allow ourselves to be awestruck by nature. Laird Hamilton explains, "When you get yourself into nature—in all its majesty, volume, and power—you are put into a position of insignificance very quickly. As you're now at the bottom of the pecking order, you're able to properly assess what you're doing. There's a certain level of humility that nature demands of you, especially when you're fully participating in it. That puts you in the perfect mind-set to be truly conscious."[49]

I'm not saying you should never post a picture of your new and improved physique. You should get praise if you've worked your ass off (sometimes literally) and achieved something you never thought possible. What I'm advocating is to have a better, conscious relationship between exercise and your body.

So if looking at pictures of people with amazing physiques on the internet motivates you to train, make sure you want to emulate those people for the right reasons. But if such photos depress or discourage you, then stop viewing them; it's a bad habit that might be weighing on your psyche more than you realize.

Observers, Not Participants

Our culture has elevated celebrities to godlike status and obsesses over their relationships, style choices, and just about every other aspect of their lives. But it's not just the everyday happenings of the rich and famous that fascinate us. We're also fixated on what's happening with everyone we know. There are no boundaries for appropriate self-disclosure when you can live blog every moment of your existence on multiple social platforms, from anywhere and at any time.

One of the reasons that journalists like George Plimpton and Cal Fussman became so popular is that their participant journalism took us inside a story and made us feel like we were involved in it. Social media has made us all observers of other people's stories to the degree that we cease to be an active part of our own narrative. We've become a society of voyeurs.

From a health standpoint, it'd be a useful exercise (pun intended) to take note of how much time we spend on social-media sites looking into other people's lives and then compare this with the daily movement stats our fitness trackers provide. I think we'd realize that most of us put a lot more effort into online nosiness than we do into improving our own wellness and performance. Doing a media fast one day a week, on the weekend, or even for an entire week can provide a reset button. It'd be even better if we spent the time we got back on being active outdoors with our friends, spouse, or kids.

If you're concerned or anxious about cutting the cord for a certain period of time, ask yourself what you'll really miss if you do. The chances are that the honest answer is "nothing." If a week sounds impossible, then try a weekend, or start by limiting yourself to checking your social feeds only once a day, at a certain time. Set rules for restricting or removing device use during meals, first thing in the morning, and last thing at night, and follow Joe Rogan's lead by putting your phone in airplane mode when you exercise. See Tom Cooper's book *Fast Media/Media Fast: How to Clear Your Mind and Invigorate Your Life in an Age of Media Overload* for more tips.

Don't Ski for Instagram, Ski for You

In December 2015, *Outside* writer Joe Jackson wrote a guide for not looking dorky on the ski hill. Tip number four was "Don't ski for Instagram, ski for you." I'd argue that skiing, or doing any activity, for that matter, just so a friend can take cool photos of you or so you can capture GoPro footage from a weird angle completely defeats the point of skiing, snowboarding, or whatever. In this instance, the selfie taker's goal is not to move, perform, or have fun. It's to promote themselves and get validation that they're living a fun, adventure-filled life with all their followers and Facebook pseudofriends.

In the wonderful parody video "Instagram Husband," produced by the comedy group The Mystery Hour, one woman tells her husband, who's reluctant to take yet another picture of her, "But babe, we need to show the world we enjoy our lives together." Why? If we want to delight in each other's company and do exciting things, we should appreciate these moments without this artificial need to record them or asking others to validate them with likes, retweets and such. When it comes to health and performance, we need to try to focus fully on the experiences we go through to learn, progress, and reach our goals, without the distraction and anxiety of figuring out how to memorialize them digitally. Ski for you, not for Instagram.

Workouts with Friends

Competing in virtual head-to-head competitions via an app can keep indoor workouts fun when the weather sucks or you've stayed late at the office and it's dark outside. But what about when it's a 70-degree, cloudless summer day and you're still choosing to row, cycle, or run that 10k against online "friends" instead of going outside to do the same with real friends— you know, those people who got you into your chosen sport and whom you actually know? In this case, the promise of online community is actually breeding isolation instead of real interaction. Not to mention the fact that some companies are now touting their product's ability to let you taunt others, and somehow think this fits in the "inspire" section of their glossy marketing. If you find you're spending more time racing and training with semianonymous people online than you are with true friends and family members, then maybe you need to put some more effort into the latter. In this case, you really *do* need to get out more.

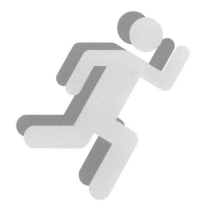

Laird Hamilton knows the importance of forging unbreakable bonds with friends in some of the most extreme conditions on the planet. When he was pioneering tow-in surfing with Dave Kalama, Brett Lickle, Darrick Doerner, and the rest of the Strapped Crew in the biggest swells ever surfed, the responsiveness of whoever was manning the Jet Ski and safety sled in the channel was the difference between living and dying. When I asked Laird about the brotherhood these experiences forged, he told me, "Community is really where we belong and that's how we evolved. When you have that and you're in nature together with someone, that's when we're at our apex. Sometimes the environment is demanding our camaraderie in order to survive because of its extremity. But there's also value in just sharing the beauty of a rainbow. I believe there's a spiritual aspect as well when you're with your friends in the water. As the biblical saying goes, 'When two or more are gathered in my name, there shall I be.'"[50]

The Parable of the Wearables Widow

One of the promises of fitness technology is that it builds community and brings people together. This might be true for some people, but for many others, fixation on fitness and the technology that furthers it ends up doing just the opposite. Instead of spending time on building and maintaining real relationships, some fanatics are rerouting their energy into checking their stats, comparing data with friends, and looking at leaderboards to see how high they rank. This stats obsession has created a new phenomenon: the wearables widow (and widower).

Here's how *Wired* contributor Jeff Foss describes an incident in Rocky Mountain National Park that made him realize how far gone he was: "I was carrying my 14-month-old son on my back, and I suddenly caught myself not only tracking our progress (there's a hiking mode) but also pausing and unpausing the app every time we stopped to inspect a wildflower or wave at a marmot. For this I was duly scolded by my wife, and I began to think more critically about my relationship with tracking. The more I attempted to track every minute, it seemed, the less engaged I became from the moment."[51]

It doesn't have to be this way. Fortunately, there are some apps out there—and others coming down the pike—that are designed to encourage authentic community, rather than destroy it. One of the reasons that I started building training programs for former Twitter CEO Dick Costolo's Chorus is that I believe in the platform's potential in this regard. Let's hope that the technology he's building will help reverse the trend of mapping runs, bike rides, and other endeavors turning into relationship-starving obsessions.

The New Age of Accountability

While social-media use can quickly morph into obsession and narcissism, some online activities can help people reach their health goals. Sherry Page and others from the University of Massachusetts Medical School found that people who started a weight-loss blog lost an average of 42.3 pounds if they posted regular (read: not crazy, minute-by-minute) updates and stuck with their blog for several months.[52] Facebook, Instagram, and other social-media sites could provide similar benefits, provided you're using them as accountability tools to help encourage you to reach a goal, rather than as opportunities for brag-fests about how ripped you're looking.

Or, if you're not just vainly searching for validation, you can use social media as a useful motivational tool. Having trouble sticking to a workout program? Try posting on Facebook and tagging friends who you know are highly motivated. Ask them to help you stay on track. Let them know you'll be posting about your workout every day (or five times a week, or whatever your goal is) and want them to bust your chops if you skip a day. You could take it a step further and say that if you fail to meet a one-month goal, you'll give each member of the accountability group ten bucks. I'm sure you'll find plenty of takers.

Doesn't She Have Any Mates?

As Mick "Crocodile" Dundee, Aussie actor Paul Hogan had many memorable lines. One of the best comes in response to the revelation that his crush, Sue, regularly meets with a psychiatrist to talk about her problems. Dumbfounded, Mick responds, "Doesn't she have any mates?" Maybe we should start asking ourselves the same question when it comes to our fitness. One company promises that its virtual assistant will provide you with motivational text messages throughout the day, "like a friend." If you need some extra accountability and motivation to meet your goals, my suggestion would be to forget the app and find a *real* friend to train with and offer mutual encouragement.

As Brad Stulberg wrote in an insightful story on this topic, "It's a lot harder to ignore a training partner than it is to ignore a wrist strap."[53] To make the most of your partnership, set certain training goals together periodically and decide how often you're going to work out and how long each session should last. Look at your calendars and find mutually convenient times for working out that you know you can stick to, whether that's when you get home from the office or early in the morning. Also establish how many times a week you're going to work out together, and be realistic about blackout days when you know your kids have activities or you have date night with your significant other.

A Culture of Obsession

It's all too easy to see obsession in our society. We're fixated on our sports teams, our favorite brands, the exercises we prefer and the diets we follow. We're even obsessed with ourselves: how we look and what we're able to do. And, of course, we're obsessed with technology.

Who's Your Tribe?

One of the reasons that people flock to stadiums and bars to watch their favorite team play each week is that team sports offers the kind of tribal affiliations that six million years of evolution have taught us we need to survive. That's why we buy all-access cable TV packages, join fantasy leagues, and clothe ourselves and our kids in brightly colored jerseys—not to mention hating those people over there because that red gear they're wearing means they're our archrivals. Over the past few years, we've seen the same kind of tribalism become more prevalent in certain fitness movements and among adherents to specific brands. It's not enough to just wear the t-shirt and put the bumper sticker on your car. You're also expected to buy in wholesale to their training philosophy and mock all other, lesser systems. If you're part of their in-group, you need to eat the way they do, too. This is the new dogmatism.

It's not just fitness brands that are getting in on the tribal action; device and app providers are, too. If you're wearing a certain type of wearable, you're one of "us" now, like the devotees of the omniscient social media platform in the film *The Circle*, whom Tom Hanks's character calls his "Circlers." Online mapping and tracking apps inspire similar levels of fanaticism and often have their own lexicon that each newbie should be given a cheat sheet to decode. Some might say that what we're looking at here is a community that creates a sense of belonging, which is valid for certain people who know how to keep their membership of a particular fitness tribe in check. The issue is that many can't help but become zealots and let their participation morph into a cultlike, brainwashed adherence to every point in the handbook.

I've seen enough of this phenomenon from the inside to know that such tribalism is not only exclusionary and cliquey but can also become extremely unhealthy. There's nothing wrong with feeling an affinity to a sport or group, but how much fun is it to be around friends who can talk of nothing but the supreme awesomeness of their latest fitness fad?

When complete devotion to an organization or product starts to become bigger than anything else in your life, it's time to take a step back and look at what that means for your relationships, your family life, and your own individuality. Sticking to a system chapter and verse vastly limits your potential for exploration and growth, and letting a certain technology dominate your thinking and actions leads all too quickly down a path on which your decisions are no longer your own.

You Are More Than Your Race Results

One of the pitfalls of going all-in with a certain sport is that you can come to a place where your entire identity is wrapped up in your performance. We often see this on social media— the friend who only posts about her latest cycling exploits or the cousin who seems fixated on how much he's lifting in the gym each day. When it comes to competitive or pro athletes, limiting your sense of self-worth to your training and race results is a dangerous game that you lose each time you fall short of your own expectations. Lenny Wiersma has

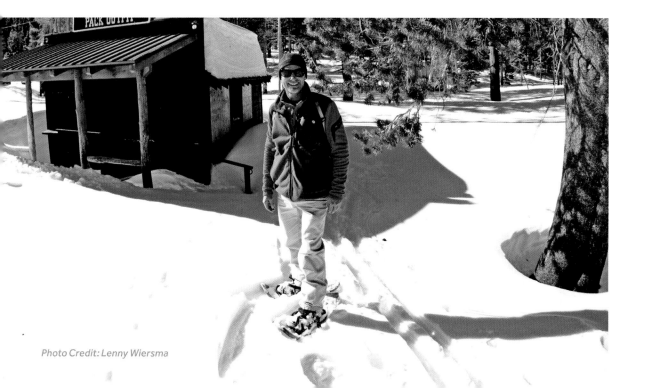

Photo Credit: Lenny Wiersma

seen this play out with Olympians time and time again but believes there's a simple antidote: "The athletes who have the healthiest perspectives are those that have a broad range of interests outside their sport and other hobbies," he said. "They're often the ones who have the most engaged fans, too, because we want our athletes to be real people we can relate to."

So even if you're an accomplished competitor, you might want to assess how many of your posts relate to your sport, what you're projecting to the world, and how this impacts how you view yourself. If you see that your self-worth has become dictated by your results, try to reassess your own standards and introduce new interests that broaden your perspective on life.

Does This Shirt Make My Arms Look Small?

When we think of image-related disorders, the first to come to mind are those that are eating-related, like bulimia and anorexia. These are obviously very serious and pervasive conditions, yet they're not the only problems of this type. There are also conditions in which people who are big and strong see a hollowed-out, puny reflection when they look in a mirror. This is one example of a condition known in the medical community as body dysmorphic disorder, and it cannot fail to be perpetuated by the selfies that other musclemen and women continually post. It might be an extreme example, but looking at the latest pics or vintage shots of Arnold Schwarzenegger is enough to give anyone an inferiority complex. If you can draw inspiration from Arnie or someone else who has what you consider to be the perfect physique, that's great. But as VitalityPro cofounder Dr. Frank Merritt says, "They should inspire you not to become them but to become the best version of you."[54]

It's also self-destructive to constantly compare yourself to the looks of celebrities or stats of pro athletes. Competition is beneficial in many ways, but when we're focusing on either the aesthetics—looking like the latest Hollywood action star, say—or the performance—like the one-rep maxes of your favorite football player—of others who you won't actually be competing against, you're chasing the unobtainable and will only end up disappointed and probably injured.

It's not just beach and gym photos of actors and athletes that can become harmful. Some world-class competitors post videos of themselves doing crazy exercises and workouts that they can get away with because of their proficiency but that are far beyond the reach of the average person. In our culture of celebrity obsession, we think, "Well if so-and-so is doing this, I need to be doing it, too," and try to replicate their exploits. Maybe we even post pictures of ourselves emulating our heroes and heroines—right before we tear a muscle, slip a disc, or drop that ludicrously heavy weight on ourselves. While we need to push ourselves and test our capabilities, imitating elite athletes is not the way to go about it, particularly when they're doing exercises that can be a one-way ticket to the office of your chiropractor, physical therapist, or orthopedic surgeon.

Tech + Exercise = Addiction Amplified

Though studies find that most people buy wearables to try to improve their health, our activity trackers and smartwatches soon become yet another way to obsessively check our e-mail and send and receive texts every few minutes. One survey found that the typical American touches his or her phone 2,617 times a day, and that's not taking into account the additional interactions people have with their fitness-related devices.[55] Several companies advertise their wearables' communication features by reassuring you that if you buy their e-mail– and texting-enabled device you "won't miss out." On a message, maybe. But you may lose something else if you turn on this function and are texting and e-mailing while exercising. How is *that* going to improve your workout or, more importantly, the learning you should gain from it?

Though *Washington Post* columnist Mark Smith had some positive things to report while wearing three activity trackers for a year, he also admitted that there were many downsides, including constant notifications: "The watch, in tandem with the phone in my pocket and the wearables on my other wrist, have allowed me to become part machine. Digital information now courses through me, delivered in deliberate and learned sets of vibrations."[56] So the external validation that someone (or something, if it's a company's automated e-mail system) wants to interact with us via e-mail is now not only visual or audible but also tactile. And yet many people can go a day, a week, or longer with little to no actual human touch.

Smith's colleague Nora Krug decided to ditch the technology when she realized that "data and music had become a crutch." After reverting to tech-free outdoor swims, yoga sessions, and runs, she told her readers, "I'm beginning to miss the technology less and less. I can hear my breath and the sound of my feet. I am more aware of how my body is moving and of the cars and dogs along the path. Birds provide the music. And just because I don't record my workouts for posterity, it doesn't mean they don't count. In fact, they matter even more."[57]

The New Neediness

The maker of the sensor-equipped tennis racket that we mentioned earlier promises users "a special badge for each new improvement." One popular app now offers a virtual trophy case to "showcase your accomplishments." This is the same kind of operant conditioning psychologist B. F. Skinner experimented with and that we use when we give our kids gold stars for doing their chores. While there's nothing diabolical about fitness trackers offering buzzes, beeps, and badges, the idea that we seek such rewards from a machine does make me wonder how needy we're becoming.

Positive reinforcement can be a very effective coaching tool if used discerningly, but if we get gold stars for every little milestone, we're being rewarded for mediocrity rather than real achievement. From a neuroscience standpoint, we're creating a feedback loop in our brains that gives us a little squirt of dopamine and other "happy hormones" each time we earn another gold star. This is ingraining a habit that encourages us to keep doing a little more each day, even when this becomes detrimental and what we really need to progress is to do a little less, but better and more skillfully. If you don't want to completely give up the extrinsic rewards your fitness technology offers, you can break the habit loop by not using it a day or two each week. Or better yet, get with a friend who's a similarly dedicated user and agree to quit together for a month. Going cold turkey might seem daunting, but having that accountability will help you stay strong.

Kicking the Habit: Replacing External Reinforcement with Internal Purpose

I've know a lot of people who panic when they're not wearing their fitness tracker because they believe their efforts while unplugged won't count. This means they've come to believe that unless their effort is being measured and recorded, it's worthless. There are even social media hashtags—like #stravafail—dedicated to this.[58] Such people also fall into the trap of thinking that if they don't accumulate more today— more reps, more rounds, more laps—then they've failed. This is a dangerous game to play, physically and emotionally. Such a mind-set suggests a deep overdependence on a device and some troubling self-worth issues, which technology is merely exacerbating.

So what happens when someone tries to go cold turkey and shoves their tracker in a drawer or deletes their monitoring apps? Not surprisingly, they go through withdrawal symptoms. "Transitioning from the quantified self back to the regular old self can be a long, grueling mental process," wrote Cari

Romm in *New York Magazine*'s August 26, 2016, issue. After ditching her wearable, she felt "a weird sense of nihilism that's been dogging me the past five days—the feeling that walking doesn't matter, that all my uncounted steps are somehow for naught. It's not enough that they get me to where I'm going; they don't have the meaning they used to."[59]

Romm goes on to cite a study by Jordan Etkin from Duke University, who found that when people unplug, they do less of their chosen activity than when they were tracking it. So if you're removing the external motivation that such a device provides, what do you replace it with? The answer is to rediscover the very thing that hooked you on your sport from the get-go: the challenge of self-improvement, the joy of discovery, and the pleasure of the activity itself. Sometimes when we defer to a wearable it switches our focus to competition, so that the activity itself is no longer enough and we can't enjoy a pickup basketball game or a company softball league without worrying about our stats. "Love of the game" might be a cliché, but it's also a valid phrase that reminds us what pure motivation and enjoyment look like.

When I talked to Lenny Wiersma, sports psychologist for USA Swimming and the UCLA swimming and water polo teams, about this topic, he told me that fitness trackers can be fine for early-stage motivation, but then said that he isn't sure if wearables will keep people in the game long enough to see the changes they want. So if they're not going to derive benefit from self-monitoring past a certain point, what can they do to keep active? Replace an external motivator with an internal one that's combined with being outdoors.

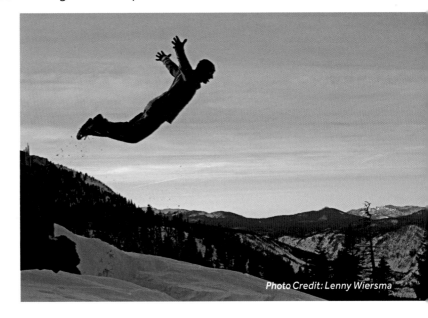

Photo Credit: Lenny Wiersma

"If you look at surfers, snowboarders, and other extreme sports athletes, nature is a large part of why they keep doing an activity that involves danger and risk," he said.

Initially they get a rush and try to replicate that, but eventually their motivation shifts. Being in a natural environment forces us to be present and conscious of what's happening. So much of our life does not require us to do that. In his film *The Fourth Phase,* Travis Rice said he's no longer going to be helicoptered onto a peak because he wants to be able to know the mountain well enough to climb it before he descends. The only way he's going to do that is to ascend the mountain on his own, even though it might take a week to summit and he might then snowboard down in a matter of minutes. But his driving force is now learning more about the environment he's performing in.[60]

You might not be carving new powder on a mountainside like Travis, but you can enrich your exercise experiences by finding new activities that are fun and are difficult or impossible to quantify. If you're a numbers person who still needs to get a simple quantification fix, then just set a goal related to the frequency of such an activity, like, "I'm going to surf three times a week this summer."

Anxious and Baffling Times

We're living in a constant state of high anxiety. From the fear-driven television news we watch to the alarmism of political bloggers to the fear of missing out that perpetuates our need to update others on our every action and simultaneously look at theirs, so much of our environment is making us twitchy. The trouble is that our body doesn't know the difference between real and perceived threats when it comes to stress and the negative, multisystemic effects it has on inflammation, the pituitary-adrenal axis, and so much more. As Dave Asprey writes in *Head Strong,* many of us are in "a constant state of emergency."[61]

Constantly monitoring our bodies is heightening our anxiety even more. As *Wired* contributor Jon Mooallem put it in a March 2017 article about how wearables often strain relationships, we can quickly become bedeviled by "the cycle of incentivizing and disincentivizing, of judgment and anxiety, afflicting you: that feeling that you can never take enough steps or unlock enough REM sleep."[62] How many times have you thrown up your hands during a frustrating day and said something like, "I *have* to work out tonight"? Movement is supposed to provide a release valve for the stresses of our crowded, overstimulating busy days. So why do we make the very thing that's meant to be calming and cathartic into yet another stressor by continually looking down at our wrists to check our pace and progress?

As anxious as wearables can make us when they're attached to us, some argue that we're even more worried if we have to do without them for any length of time after we're hooked. In an insightful article for *Inc.,* Howard Tullman wrote, "If you don't believe this [addiction to activity trackers] is a problem here and now, just see how you react when you discover midday that you forgot to sufficiently charge your device and it's no longer measuring your activity. We've all experienced the angst associated with our mobile phones dying, but this is even worse. And, if you really want to go 'cold turkey' just see how hard it is to put your device on the bed stand one morning and try to 'leave home without it.' I don't think you can do it."[63]

I completely agree with Tullman's premise here, but I believe that you can actually go wearables-free for a day or two, and, for the sake of your stress levels and overall health, you *must,* at least once in a while. If you do, try to be mindful of your mental and emotional state during planned workouts and normal movement-related activities, like walking to the mailbox or around your office building. I'll wager that once you

Searching for Stillness

One of the antidotes to the poison of tech-induced anxiety is to disconnect and get out in nature for long enough that you start to feel comfortable not checking your activity score or calories-burned total. Here's Lenny Wiersma with a profound case study.

Every summer I take a couple of backpacking trips. I met a neighbor while out walking my dog and after we got to know each other a little, asked him if he'd like to come too. He was really excited about it, even though he'd never been camping or slept in a tent. On the seven-hour drive to Mount Whitney he was checking his phone almost constantly. The first couple of days he seemed worried. But then on day three I noticed a real change in him. He started becoming more confident and peaceful. I bumped into him a few months after the trip and asked him how he was doing. He told me, "There's not a day that goes by when I don't think about Whitney or draw from that experience we shared." It wasn't just the five days it took to get to the back side of the mountain or the time it took to summit and come back down. Deep immersion in nature had a lasting effect on him.[64]

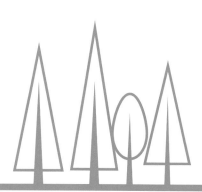

overcome the discomfort of not having your device on your wrist, you'll feel calmer and less anxious. Once you get to this point, put the wearable back on, try it again for a couple of days, and compare how you feel. If you prefer having it back then keep it around, but if you feel worse than during your trial separation, maybe it's time to consider a permanent breakup.

Take the Nature Challenge

When Andy moved from central Indiana to Southern California to take a position at California State University, Fullerton, he soon found that despite being in a climate that's more conducive to being outside, he was actually getting outdoors less because of his research and teaching schedule. So he came up with an easy way to solve this problem: doing tasks that usually kept him in the office outdoors. Andy bought headphones that had a microphone and started walking around campus to take all his calls. Rather than having student-adviser meetings in his office, he met the student somewhere outdoors and re-created the Steve Jobs walking meeting, which also had the benefit of giving himself and these students more movement in their day. Our friend Doug Larson, who's one of Andy's copresenters on the *Barbell Shrugged* podcast, does something similar, getting up earlier than his wife and son so he can take his laptop out on the back patio and get some work done while he watches the sun rise. He then joins his family for breakfast with a clear mind, knowing that he's gotten ahead of what would've been a jam-packed morning.

An Open-Sourced Life

Jocko Willink, former Navy SEAL and coauthor of the excellent book *Extreme Ownership,* said that over the course of his military career he came to appreciate that "discipline equals freedom."[65] When it comes to being active in nature, discipline means creating a daily rhythm of purposeful practice in activities that intrigue, excite, and challenge us, and being open to new experiences as well. Creating such a mind-set frees us from the boundaries of relying on technology, always being indoors, and closing off our world, and reopens us to the possibilities of infinite progress that exists when we live fully and deeply. We've been given the gift of life—we need to live it!

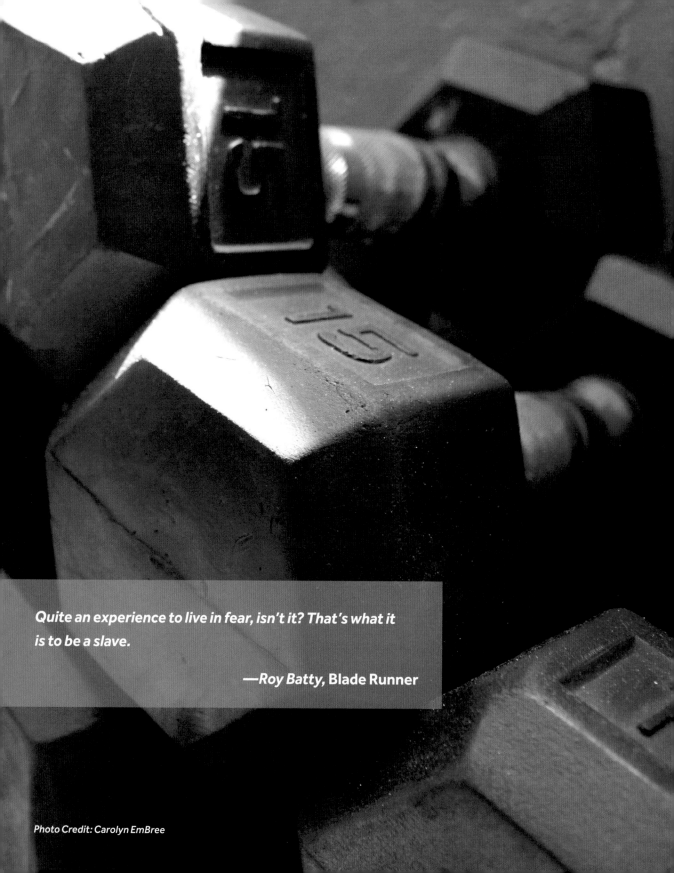

Quite an experience to live in fear, isn't it? That's what it is to be a slave.

—*Roy Batty*, Blade Runner

Photo Credit: Carolyn EmBree

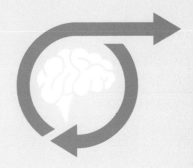

CHAPTER 3
CIRCUIT-BREAKING THE STRESS CYCLE

From childhood, we're taught that the faster and harder we push ourselves, the further ahead we're going to get—in our jobs, with the possessions we acquire, and in our health. We've also come to accept that technology plays a crucial part in this progressive plan, which will someday lead us to some kind of utopia. So we've created a world that's always switched on and always on the go.

The trouble is that we're lying to ourselves if we think that there are no downsides to this approach. My friend (and Frank Merritt's VitalityPro colleague) Brandon Rager reminded me recently that when we're always available, we feel obliged to answer every call, reply to every text, and like every social-media post that comes our way. In doing so, we take time away from our friends and families and reinforce an exaggerated sense of obligation. Because we can access our work e-mail in-boxes and documents from anywhere and on any device, we also feel guilty if we're not being productive around the clock. How many times have you thought, "I'd better get back to my boss on that before she thinks I'm being lazy or ignoring her"? For many of us, work-related e-mails and texts are the last things we see before we go to sleep and the first things we look at when we get up. We're bookending our days with our inflated idea of duty, guilt, and must-do-more.

Then we add in our fitness-tracking devices and apps, which, according to the most recent surveys, most people keep on them at all times, except when they're charging them. If you walk down a busy street in any city now, you not only see people looking down at their phones but have to dodge those who are checking their numbers on a wearable.

The first step in freeing ourselves is to set better boundaries. While it's admittedly difficult to do at first, you should declare certain times of the day to be tech-free zones in which you don't respond to texts, don't look at e-mails or social media, and stop checking your fitness stats. From a lifestyle perspective, it'd also be beneficial to let people know that you're not available after a certain time in the evening and before a certain time in the morning. You do not owe it to anyone (let alone any piece of technology) to be permanently connected and contactable.

In addition to periodically switching out digital days for analog ones, you should also apply the same methodology to your training. A few times a month, try exchanging your high-tech workout for an outdoor one (more on this in chapter 9).

If you usually head straight for the stepper in the gym, go run some stairs in a local stadium instead or go for a hike. Forgo your spin class for intervals around your neighborhood on your old beach cruiser or your kid's five-speed bike that's been gathering dust in the garage for a decade. Or buy a cheap sandbag and lug it around the park in place of your usual weights routine. Yes, the exact work done during all of these options is much more difficult to quantify in your spreadsheet or app if you're doing unplugged outdoor sessions, but that's fine. You should be working toward feeling better, not just improving your numbers, anyway.

The Cost of Plugging In

We're learning more and more about the clinical, psychological, and cognitive effects of being constantly connected. We joke about short attention spans and the lengths we go to in order to reach the goal our app has set, but there's an unnerving grain of truth in those jokes: we're changing the way our brains work and making ourselves more anxious than ever.

What Was That? The Plague of Continuous Partial Attention

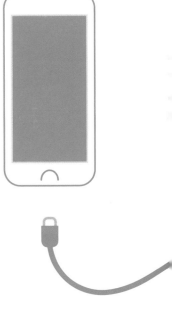

It's not a stretch to say that our lives have never been more fragmented or distracted. Uninterrupted access to millions of websites, the ability to send messages around the world in the blink of an eye, and carrying around a productivity tool / music player / camera / communication device plus a wearable with us wherever we go means that we're never bored. And this is precisely the problem.

Because we have so much going on at all times, we can never fully immerse ourselves in anything. In the age of perpetual stimulation and distraction, we've become so scatterbrained that technology thought leader Linda Stone coined the phrase *continuous partial attention* (CPA). Stone explains it as "an always-on, anywhere, anytime, any place behavior that involves an artificial sense of constant crisis. We are always on high alert when we pay continuous partial attention. . . . In a 24/7, always-on world, continuous partial attention used as our dominant attention mode contributes to a feeling of overwhelm, over-stimulation and to a sense of being unfulfilled. We are so accessible, we're inaccessible. The latest, greatest powerful technologies have contributed to our feeling increasingly powerless."[66]

CPA doesn't just apply to social media or our work lives but also to how we exercise. If you're a member of a gym, how often do you see someone taking a call or texting while they're on a cardio machine, or stopping a lifting session to take a self-promoting selfie in the mirror? Doing so denies us the mind-clearing release that focused physical activity promises and means we derive less physiological benefit from the time and effort we put into exercising. And as Stone says, something that could help us feel empowered in fact leaves us feeling more powerless than ever.

Athletic Obsessive Compulsive Disorder

If you read widely, you've probably come across stories warning about the ill effects of checking e-mail dozens of times a day, constantly posting updates to social-media sites, and getting involved in perpetual texting conversations. Yet very few people have explored how our attempts to become completely self-quantified are contributing to the constant sense of unease that many of us feel.

Spend enough time around elite athletes and you'll see that the phenomenon of health anxiety is all too real. Counting calories, measuring power output, logging sets and reps . . . In any other sphere, these would be viewed as the hallmarks of obsessive-compulsive disorder! Yet in the world of sports, such habits are not merely overlooked but actually encouraged by coaches who are just as fixated on metrics as their athletes.

In our mission to be fitter and perform better, it's very easy to go to extremes and lose all sense of moderation. If you're moving most of the day and eating predominantly whole, unprocessed foods, you really need to stop recording every calorie and gram of fat, sugar, or protein, and you shouldn't be relying on an app to estimate the healthiness or unhealthiness of each meal and snack. By following a basic 80/20 approach to activity and nutrition—eight out of ten times you make good decisions—that scoop of ice cream you enjoy once in a while is not going to kill you or prevent you from reaching your goals. Neither should you try to push through an injury or illness to make sure you reach some app-supplied daily target. Doing so is just going to mean that you face a longer layoff. You know it's a bad idea to work out when every system in your body is screaming for you to rest. You just have to start listening to yourself again and stop waiting for a piece of technology to tell you that it knows best.

Downshifting

For many of us, working out and being active is our stress relief. It helps us forget about work and family problems for a while and lets us physically relax (at least eventually)—or so we assume. Unfortunately, it's not always that easy. We can have trouble downshifting after intense activity, and we can create both physical and psychological stress *through* our workouts. De-stressing is crucial but is becoming increasingly difficult because we rarely disconnect and make a conscious effort to do what yoga expert Jill Miller suggests and "turn on our off switch." In fact, many of us don't even know how to do this, or why technology is making downshifting more difficult than ever.

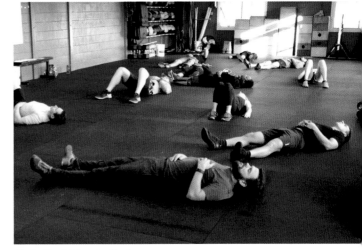

Photo Credit: Carolyn EmBree

The Hunt and the Nap

When they're hunting or playing, animals go all-out and then lie down to rest or nap immediately. Male lions take this pattern to the extreme, sleeping up to twenty hours a day. The key here isn't the amount of time spent resting but the way that a wild predator, or even your pets, can go from running and jumping at full speed to relaxation in moments. Contrast this to our inability to downshift adequately after activity. We're really good at using caffeine, warm-ups, and pre-workout supplements to fire us up, but we're very bad at dowsing the flames. That five-minute cooldown you (maybe) do after your fitness class or run? Not going to cut it.

In his fantastic book *Why Zebras Don't Get Ulcers,* Robert Sapolsky states that we're looking at the relationship between exercise and stress all wrong. "We've been focusing on the stress-related consequences of activating the cardiovascular system too often," he writes. "What about turning it off at the end of each psychological stressor? If you are turning on the sympathetic nervous system all the time, you're chronically shutting off the parasympathetic. And this makes it more difficult to slow things down, even during those rare moments when you're not feeling stressed about something."[67]

So what can we do to go from a state of high alert during exercise into parasympathetic recovery—that is, to go from the high-alert fight-or-flight state into a rest-and-digest mode? One thing is to incorporate breathing into an extended cooldown, which should consist of five to fifteen minutes of slow activity, such as walking, and a couple of mobility exercises that target the major muscle groups you just stimulated. Kelly Starrett's book *Becoming a Supple Leopard;* his website, MobilityWOD; and his YouTube channel have all you need on this topic.

While you're doing this cooldown and mobility work, focus on returning your breathing to normal. Take a deep, slow breath in from your diaphragm, which means your belly should expand more than your chest. Then take even more time on the exhale, letting yourself deflate like a balloon, as my friend, colleague, and breathing guru Wim Hof says. Take at least fifteen breaths like this, then do a single inhale hold (breathe in and hold for as long as you can without passing out!) and then a single exhale hold.

Sapolsky explains why long exhales help you downshift from a stress state into one of relaxation and restoration: "When you exhale, the parasympathetic half turns on, activating your vagus nerve in order to slow things down (this is why many forms of meditation are built around extended exhalations)."[68] For those who've never done this type of breathing before, some fitness trackers and smartwatches now offer a breath-guiding function that can show you the way the first few times. Again, I'd encourage you to concentrate on your breathing itself, and notice how the breath cycle slows your heart rate down. Once your device or app has shown you the way, try to do without it and let sensation be your guide. If you can't reproduce what you think you've learned on your own, with no technology and nobody to guide you, then you haven't really mastered the skill and need to practice it more. Use the device or app once again and pay even closer attention to yourself, then put it away and retest. Repeat as necessary until you've got it down.

Stress Rx: *Not* More Stress

In our app-driven quest for more, more, more, we've unwittingly added yet another stressor into our lives that threatens to tip some of us over the edge. We go from a stressful work environment to a gym and do a stressful workout, then head home to a stressful family environment, believing incorrectly that the thirty minutes or hour of frantic activity has helped us de-stress. Add in the fact that many gyms subject us to loud, unrelenting music and more TVs than you'd find in the average sports bar, and you have a full-on sensory assault that is far more demanding than all but the most extreme of stress-inducing jobs. Then we realize that we're two thousand steps short of our daily target, so we go out for a run later that night, or else dwell on how we've fallen short of our wearables' expectations yet again.

In strength training, we recognize the need to include rest periods in our sessions because the body needs time to recover from the last set and rebound for the next one. We also know that it's the recovery time after exercise that leads to adaptation, not the activity itself (this doesn't just apply to lifting weights but to any kind of sport or exertion). Frank Merritt made the good point that you cannot carry a two-hundred-pound weight above your head all day; it'd crush you.[69] Yet we've created a lifestyle that demands us to do just that in terms of other stressors. And unfortunately, the body doesn't distinguish between the type of load you're placing on it. Stress is stress, and when there's no respite for weeks, months, or years, we can only expect grave consequences (pun intended).

Lenny Wiersma conducted an oral interview–based study of big-wave surfers and found that those who weren't pros used their water time to manage the stress of their jobs.

> Dr. Mark Renneker was one of the first guys to surf Mavericks and found that surfing provided this relief from his job as an oncologist that he couldn't find any other way. He juggles all these balls in the air when he goes in every day to work with cancer patients. Coming into this extreme natural environment forces you to shut everything else out. Because if your connection shifts to your job and you don't focus on the wave, you're going to get killed. If he was out in the ocean and anything from his personal or work life came into his head, he said he knew it was a significant thing he needed to pay attention to when he was done surfing because nature will only allow the truly important thoughts to get through in those moments.[70]

So, like Mark Renneker, we need to make sure that when we spend time moving, we do so in a way that provides a respite from the constant demands we're placing on ourselves from the time we get up till the time we go to bed. An obvious way is to seek out restorative immersion in nature. But on those days that we do have to exercise indoors, I suggest doing it in a way that reduces our stress load, rather than increasing it. This includes putting our devices to one side and making a conscious effort to better sense how we're moving and breathing throughout the activity.

Also try to integrate stress-busting breaks into your workday. If you're trying to brainstorm, head outside and take audio notes on your phone or voice recorder. Or take the time to walk to see a colleague in person rather than copping out and just sending them a text, e-mail, or IM. Stumped by a big project? Do your workout earlier than planned to clear your mind.

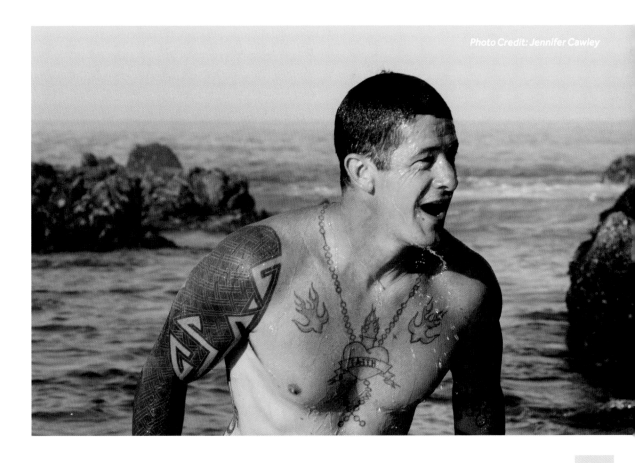

Photo Credit: Jennifer Cawley

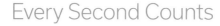

Every Second Counts

Henry Ford was obsessed with eliminating what he viewed as wasted time from his assembly line. His methods reduced the time it took to build a car from twelve hours to less than two. When the rest of the manufacturing world caught up with what Ford was doing, efficiency became the name of the game in factories across the globe. In the 1950s and 1960s, we saw management experts trying to introduce similar principles into offices. So for half a century or more, we've been conditioned by our workplace that an efficient worker is a productive worker, and therefore a good one.

With the massive advances in consumer technology over the same period, we've also tried desperately to make our lives outside of work more efficient. Why use a slow cooker when you can fire up the microwave? What's the point in going to the library when you can just download a book (maybe this one!) instantly? This mentality has also made its way into fitness. The crazy hitchhiker Ben Stiller's character picks up in *There's Something About Mary* tells him about his plan for a seven-minute abs program that will best the eight-minute version already available. He adds, "We guarantee just as good a workout as the eight-minute folks." Stiller's character agrees but then says, "Unless of course someone comes up with six-minute abs."

The humor of this scene masks an uncomfortable truth: when it comes to our health, fitness, and performance, we want to do as little as possible so we have more time in our days. We have apps that will take us through those seven-minute abs (or maybe even six), promising to give us the six-pack Hollywood has told us we need. Then we move on quickly to the next thing and the next, sure to cram as much in as possible so we don't miss out on anything.

But our fear of missing out means we *are* missing something. Actually, lots of things. Filling every second with activity is also stressing us out, which not only makes us feel anxious but also changes our physiology. We now know that continual stress can lead to adrenal fatigue and spike our blood pressure and inflammation levels, which contribute to a whole host of diseases. British philosopher Alan Watts advised, "Stop measuring days by degree of productivity and start experiencing them by degree of presence." Amen to that.

There's nothing wrong with efficiency, but when we apply our I-want-it-now approach to our health, we often end up with benefits that don't last and motivation that fades once the initial gains level off. We also forget that playing a sport well or getting better at an active pursuit like rock climbing isn't just about results, it's also the process that's beneficial. Becoming bigger, stronger, and faster (or lighter, leaner, and more cut) is not what improves your performance level—acquiring and developing skills is. And as Robert Greene puts it in his fine book *Mastery,* "When it comes to mastering a skill, time is the magic ingredient."[71] This is why, if you're going to be doing something more than a couple of times, you should abandon the shortcuts and commit to slow, steady improvement, which requires regular and complete engagement.

Slow and Steady Wins the Race

It's easy to get caught up in the idea that pushing ourselves further and harder always means better results, but when it comes to physical activity, more isn't always better. In fact,

slowing down can have benefits we often overlook: it allows you to focus on different aspects of your practice, such as endurance and technique; it helps prevent overuse injuries; and it reduces stress—both physical and psychological. Plus, you can't exercise your way out of a sedentary lifestyle with a single daily workout if it's bookended by hours of inactivity. Slow and steady movement throughout the day is important for both body and brain.

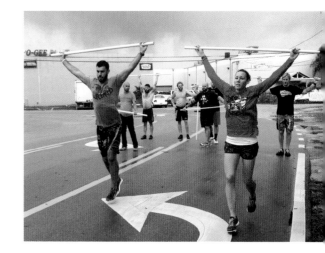

Move!

As we don't live in an agrarian society anymore and most of us aren't working on farms or in other physically demanding jobs, we've had to come up with ways to add physical activity into each day. Movement can help us start our morning positively or decompress after a jam-packed day, but we need to make sure we're also building in movement breaks in the hours in between. Exercising for one period—whether it's for thirty minutes, an hour, or longer—certainly has its benefits, but we can shortchange these and even start undoing them if we are sedentary the rest of the day. We risk becoming active couch potatoes who believe that a brief period of one-off exercise every twenty-four hours makes us bulletproof, when in fact, we can't outrun or outlift eight to ten hours of sitting.

Standing instead of sitting increases metabolic rate, eliminates sitting-based orthopedic problems like low back pain and lost hip function, and makes it easier to retain healthy positioning. But if you stand in one place, you're still likely to develop circulatory issues, get stiff ankles and feet, and have other issues. The key, as movement expert Dr. Kelly Starrett advises, is to stand instead of sit, add a fidget bar so you can get some micro-movement, or get in a set of a body-weight exercise, like push-ups or squats between phone meetings, and change positions and move frequently.

One study showed that moving for five minutes undoes most of the damage caused by sitting for an hour, which includes a 50 percent reduction in blood flow to the legs.[72] But if you replaced that sitting with standing, fidgeting, walking around while on phone meetings, you'd have a plan that's even better for you. Such a routine also benefits the brain: researchers from Texas A&M found that call center workers who were active throughout the day were 46 percent more productive than those who sat.[73] How much you move directly correlates to brain function, memory, and cognitive performance. It also directly impacts your mood and stress levels. Researchers at the University of Pittsburgh Brain

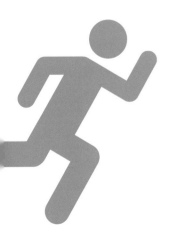

Institute found that the neural pathways engaged during movement have direct access to our brain's stress-control centers. A key to decreased stress and improved health, then, is rebooting our sedentary software and ingraining the habit of constant movement.[74]

One technology that can help in this is an app that reminds you to get up and move around at regular intervals. If you can't stand and move for most of the day, then adding movement breaks is the next best thing. Researchers at the University of Texas discovered that constant sitting makes people incapable of burning fat like those who are constantly in motion, even if they exercise intensely.[75] So move more, and when you can't, set that timer on your phone or wearable to make sure you're not sitting for long.

But don't be a slave to the app. Instead, be aware of how you feel when it goes off and you haven't been moving for a certain period of time. Do you feel sluggish or inattentive? Are you becoming restless? If so, you could use a neuro-hack (such as eating a piece of dark chocolate or playing a quick brain-training game) to complement a movement break and help you focus better when you get back to working or studying. After a while, see if you can start noticing when your attention begins to wane, your thoughts wander, or you feel sore or stiff. If you can increase your awareness to this point, you won't need the app anymore. You can also use a tool like Kelly Starrett's MWOD fidget bar to add in micro-movement that increases circulation and reduces positional fatigue.

If you have kids or grandkids, you should also try applying this thinking to them. Rather than yelling at them if they start fidgeting during their homework, encourage them to put on a song and dance around for a few minutes. They'll be much more focused when they get back to those vexing math problems or that spelling bee word list. Andy remembers being constantly told to sit still when he was growing up, but this is the exact opposite of what we should be teaching our children.

Don't Sweat It

In addition to adopting the "no pain, no gain" maxim as gospel truth, we've also convinced ourselves that for a workout to be worthwhile, we need to be sweating buckets by the end of it. I frequently do high-octane sessions by myself, with my wife, and with my athletes, but I realized long ago that you can't just hammer yourself every day. If you do, you'll end up with hormonal imbalance, poor sleep, digestive complaints, and a host of other problems, all of which are ways your body's trying to tell you that something's wrong. If you go all-out every single time you're active, your endocrine, cardiovascular, and other systems will feel like they're under constant threat and stop making positive cellular adaptations. You'll also be unable to recover adequately between sessions, and in your haste, you're more likely to abandon proper mechanics. Over time, these two factors are going to lead to injury.

Instead of trying to make sure you earn that towel you've brought with you, try varying the intensity of your sessions. When I'm working with my athletes, I call this "gearing." If your bike had eleven gears but only two of them worked properly, you'd only use those two, right? A lot of people have this issue, sticking to the gear they're most comfortable with instead of switching it up. They can maintain moderate power output for an entire 5k, but try to get them to go at maximum speed for a few one-minute intervals and they blow up. Or maybe they're fine with short, very hard efforts, but extend the work period a little at a slightly lower intensity and they fall apart.

We can all improve our gearing, and in this fast-paced, HIIT-dominated exercise climate, for many of us that means being able to slow down. Get just as comfortable moving slowly, smoothly, and rhythmically as you are going a hundred miles an hour. If you lift weights, break your technique back down to the basics with very little on the bar or even using a PVC pipe, and see where you can improve. If you can't move well with no weight while going slow, you're going to move very poorly while trying to throw around a lot of weight quickly. And whatever you do, make sure you add some more skill work before and after sessions.

From an attitude perspective, recognize that the approach that is making you sweat is also stressing you out more and that you can have a valuable experience without dripping all over the place. If your aim is to always feel exhausted at the end of every session, what you're doing is unsustainable and won't enable you to reach your goals. Instead, you should want to improve some specific aspect of your practice—whether that's power application, endurance, or skill execution—each time you exercise.

Achieving More by Doing Less

For the past decade, I've worked with an athlete who has tried to cram running marathons into her extremely hectic schedule. In addition to being a wife and mother of two children, she runs her own hairstyling business and teaches spinning classes three times a week. When we first started working together, she told me that her goal was to run a 3:30 marathon. I looked at her training logs and was horrified to see just how many miles of pavement pounding she was totaling each week. I soon made her realize that she had a naturally powerful engine and that those spinning classes were keeping her aerobic capacity topped up. Instead of trying to add yet more volume to her already maxed-out calendar (and body, for that matter), I cut her back to skill drills and three high-intensity Tabata sessions each week—that's eight sets of twenty seconds' hard effort followed by twenty seconds of active rest. Using this stripped-down program, she was able to reach her time goal and had more space in her life for her business, her family and, heaven forbid, a little relaxation.

So when I got a call from her a few months ago to say she was suffering from Achilles tendinitis—a condition she'd never had before—I knew something was amiss. She came in to see me and I asked her to be honest about her training load. Was she sticking to the program that we'd outlined together, which had worked well for so long? Sadly, no. Her tendency to do more in every area of her life had spilled over into her running, and she'd gone back to her old high-mileage ways. As a result, she not only was unable to compete in more marathons but couldn't run at all because of those aching Achilles tendons.

Now in this case, it was her personality that drove her back into an unhealthy pattern. But it's not a stretch to say that wearables and their focus on always doing a little more than yesterday can exacerbate users' excessive tendencies and feelings that they're not pushing themselves as hard as they can. We need to recognize that we can achieve more by doing less with more intent, purpose, and quality. Until then, we're going to continue seeing an increase in overuse injuries and the psychological issues that drive (and result from) doing too much, with our digital taskmasters pushing us ever onward.

What Are You Running From?

Are you punishing yourself or trying to escape a personality/psychological issue with hard workouts that you go through semiconsciously? Sometimes we can use exercise to numb ourselves from pain, sorrow, or loss, which, from the perspective of intent, is little different than drowning our sorrows in drugs or alcohol. I've known too many athletes who use running, lifting, or sports not to positively channel their emotions but to stop feeling altogether. Using exercise to escape from problems in your past, present troubles, or fears for the future doesn't eliminate the issues. It merely pushes them down deeper, meaning that when the emotional volcano erupts, it's going to do so with even greater force.

We often employ our gadgets to further desensitization and dissociation. Not only do we go through the motions of the activity, but then we spend hours obsessing over the minutiae of our performance. By burying our head in the virtual sand,

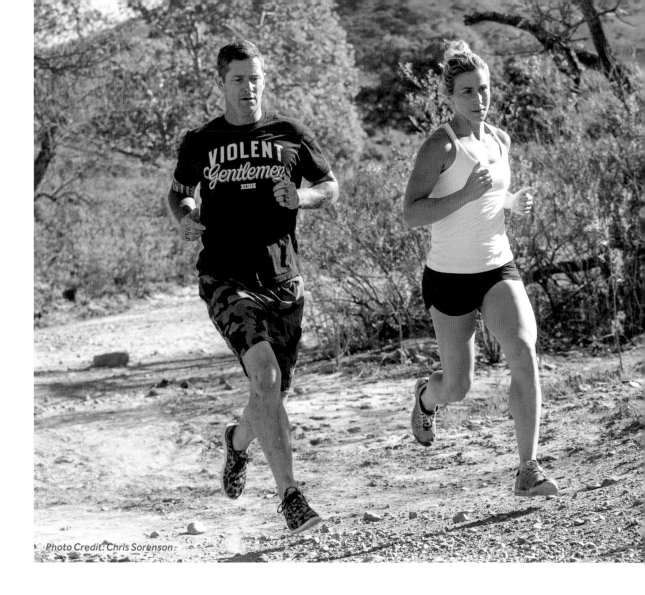

Photo Credit: Chris Sorenson

we're failing to tackle those work problems, heal a broken relationship, or confront whatever's been haunting us all these years. So we beat our bodies into submission, suppress our feelings, and tell ourselves that if we can just qualify for an Ironman, beat our PR, or reach some other milestone, everything will be alright. If this sounds familiar, you need to take off your wearable and your running shoes and pick up the phone to call a friend or family member who can help you take the first step toward shedding that baggage you're carrying.

Rest and Recovery

As important as slowing down is, it's not enough. We need *real* downtime: periods when we can let our bodies rest and recover without the stimulation of social media and the artificial light of our screens. We need high-quality, rejuvenating sleep and a lifestyle that suits our natural chronotype, whether we like to be up with the sun and asleep before ten or prefer to wake up late and stay up late. Letting our bodies and minds rest and recuperate is as important as giving them a workout.

Is Your Downtime Keeping You Up?

Read virtually any health or fitness magazine and you're likely to come across a story on the perils of overtraining. Sure, some of us are putting in way too many miles or lifting far too many pounds to let our bodies bounce back. But more often, we're not really overtraining at all but underrecovering. A big part of this issue is our evening routine. We believe that plopping down on the couch at night after a long, tiring day is in some way relaxing.

In fact, doing so has a couple of problems. The first is that it's compounding all those hours of sitting that we've already racked up and, if we exercised on the way home, undoing some of the gains that activity may have provided. The second issue, which many people are unaware of, is that watching television, checking social-media feeds, and responding to yet more e-mails is actually making us more anxious because we're being stimulated by what Dave Asprey calls "junk light." This suppresses production of melatonin, which the body needs to tell it to wind down and go to sleep. We're also flitting between multiple things when we're on our tablets, phones, or laptops, reinforcing our continuous partial attention issues and creating a sense of unease at the very time we need to feel comforted and reassured.

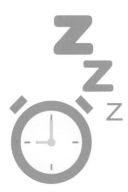

A better use of our time would be to forgo the screens for a change and dive into a good book. Reading is far more immersive than a movie or TV show and demands much greater attention than our scattered, fragmented tech-based tasks. Assuming you're sticking with hardcovers and paperbacks instead of e-books, you'll eliminate the blue light issue. You could also add in some mobility exercises, which relieve aches and pains, improve blood flow, and even, in the case of abdominal massage / gut smashing, stimulate the vagus nerve to encourage your autonomic nervous system to transition into parasympathetic recovery (see mobilitywod.com for directions).

Bad Sleep Is No Badge of Courage

Remember that episode of *Seinfeld* in which Kramer unsuccessfully tried polyphasic sleep—sleeping for multiple short periods over the course of a day—and ended up in the Hudson River trapped in a sack? This is an amusing but telling example of what happens when we don't get adequate high-quality rest. While many types of technology can make our sleep issues worse, we can put a wearable to good use in helping us quantify and qualify our slumber. Though not many studies have been conducted on the accuracy of wrist-worn devices' ability to appraise our sleep, their data collection is likely good enough to make them worth trying for this purpose.

The old-school practice of using sleep logs worked for some, but all too often we'd either forget to write down our totals, exaggerate how long we'd slept, or confuse the time that we went to bed with when we drifted off. Sleep logging also tricked us into believing that as long as we got eight hours each night, we'd leap out of bed feeling refreshed in the morning, no matter what had transpired the day before. So just like with another arbitrary eight—the number of glasses of water an adult is supposed to drink a day—we got fixated on quantity.

This obscures the reality that some people need less than eight hours and others need more, and that just as what we do each day varies, so too does our need for shut-eye. Beyond the amount of time we spend asleep, the quality of it is arguably just as important, if not more so. Say you got nine hours but were disturbed by your neighbor's dog barking, half-woken by a couple of texts because you forgot to switch off your phone notifications, and got up to use the bathroom twice. You'll likely be shocked awake by your alarm, feel groggy, and wish you could have stayed in bed for another hour or two. Contrast that to a night when you got seven hours and there were no interruptions or intrusions. You probably felt better than the morning after those unsatisfying nine hours.

Sleep is another area where we can wield technology for good and combine it with an evaluation of our mood and energy levels. You could use your fitness tracker to monitor both the quantity and, to some degree, the quality of your sleep for a week or two, using either a sleep log app or just a good old-fashioned notebook. In addition to recording what time you go to bed and wake up, it'd be helpful if you logged whether you felt okay, great, or wretched when you woke up. You could then go further and examine what you ate and drank each night, how you felt when you got into bed, and how long it took you to fall asleep. Then try to see patterns between your evening behavior, food intake, sleep quality and quantity, mood, and energy levels, both last thing at night and first thing in the morning. Once you've identified some trends, you can start making adjustments and experimenting to nail down a nighttime routine and food choices that are more conducive to a truly good night's sleep.

What's Your Sleep Score?

I have my own cautionary tale to tell about sleep tracking. A couple of years ago, I was completely burned out from working too much, and one of the side effects was disrupted sleep. It got to the point that I had to start popping prescription pills because I had no other solutions to get the rest I so desperately needed. As I started to learn more about the science of sleep, I began making changes that helped me get off the meds and on a better schedule— like replacing bright bulbs with warmer tones, eliminating electronic device exposure before I lay down, and making sure my bedroom was cold.

I figured that as part of my new sleep hygiene routine, I might as well use a sleep tracker to see if the duration and quality of my slumber had actually improved or if I was just kidding myself. The trouble is, the joke was on me. I'm a recovering hypercompetitor, and when I quantify any aspect of my life, I automatically want to beat that number. So if my "sleep score" (an arbitrary value the tracker produces using an algorithm) was a 70 that first night, I wanted at least a 72 the next time I checked, then a 74, and so on. Maybe if I really pushed myself I could reach 100!

But rather than encouraging me to form and sustain healthy habits, my desire to get a better score actually added yet another stressor. Initially, the tracker did encourage positive behavior change. I started going to bed earlier in my vain attempt to get that score up, for example. But soon enough this started creating anxiety. Eventually, I realized that tracking my sleep was not improving the quality of it and that the only number my vainglorious self-competition was increasing was my stress level. So I set the tracker aside and went back to improving my nighttime routine.

I also did some beneficial self-discovery about my chronotype (you know, night owl or early bird) and found that I do my best creative work, have my most beneficial breathing and meditation sessions, and move well in the early morning. I also became more cognizant of when I started to get tired in the evening—earlier than I'd realized. With these two insights in mind, I started going to bed earlier, not to aid my contest with a device but to improve the fit between my biorhythms and my lifestyle. I also stopped using an alarm and started getting up when I awoke, usually between 3:30 and 5:00 a.m. My wife, Erin, has the opposite chronotype and picks up speed as the day goes. So she goes to bed and wakes up later than I do. That's what works for her, and we just figure out times in the middle of the day to spend time together. I'm not saying you should be in bed at 9:00 p.m. or wake up before dawn if that doesn't jibe with your rhythms.

Nor am I saying that sleep tracking can't work for you. If you're someone who's not going to become obsessed with your sleep score, then there's no harm in using a sleep tracker. But if you're competitive, like me, it's probably not for you, and you should do a little self-exploration to find out more about your optimal sleep-wake cycle. Then experiment with tweaking your day-to-day life to better fit your chronotype, while also trying to improve your evening routine so it's more conducive to winding down instead of ramping up.

Being vs. Doing

When our identity is wrapped up in how productive we are and how many items we check off our to-do list each day, we're becoming defined by doing and have forgotten how to just be. As our calendars fill up with all kinds of commitments—from meetings and classes to kids' activities to that book club we secretly loathe—we get embroiled in a heightened version of the rat race in which we wrongly associate doing more with feeling better. In the pursuit of continual achievement, we rush headlong from one activity to the next, trying to get each one done as quickly as possible so we can cram yet more into our already overcrowded schedules. Then we spend what little free time we have left complaining about how busy we are.

What would it feel like if you just stopped? If you cleared your calendar and kept it empty for a week or two? If you did things that you wanted to do, rather than just those you felt obligated to do? It's probably hard to even conceive of such a thing. That's exactly why you should try it. And then engage fully, openly, and thankfully in the experiences you've chosen. You'll likely realize that you never want to go back to that old, chaotic, where-do-I-have-to-go-next excuse for an existence.

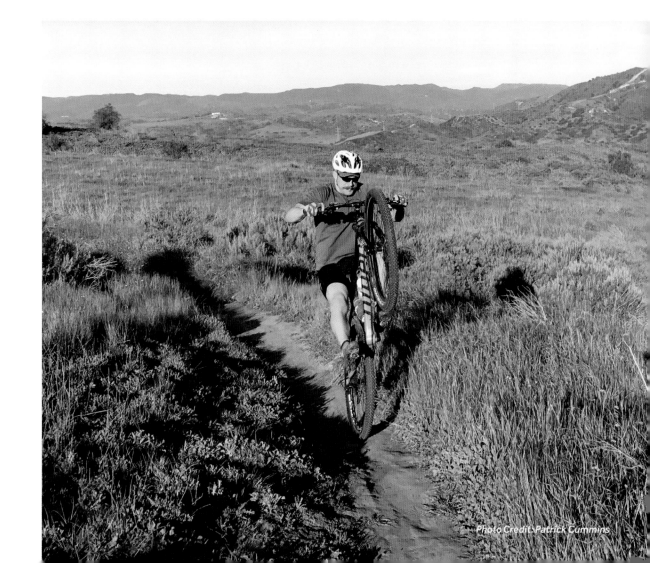

Photo Credit: Patrick Cummins

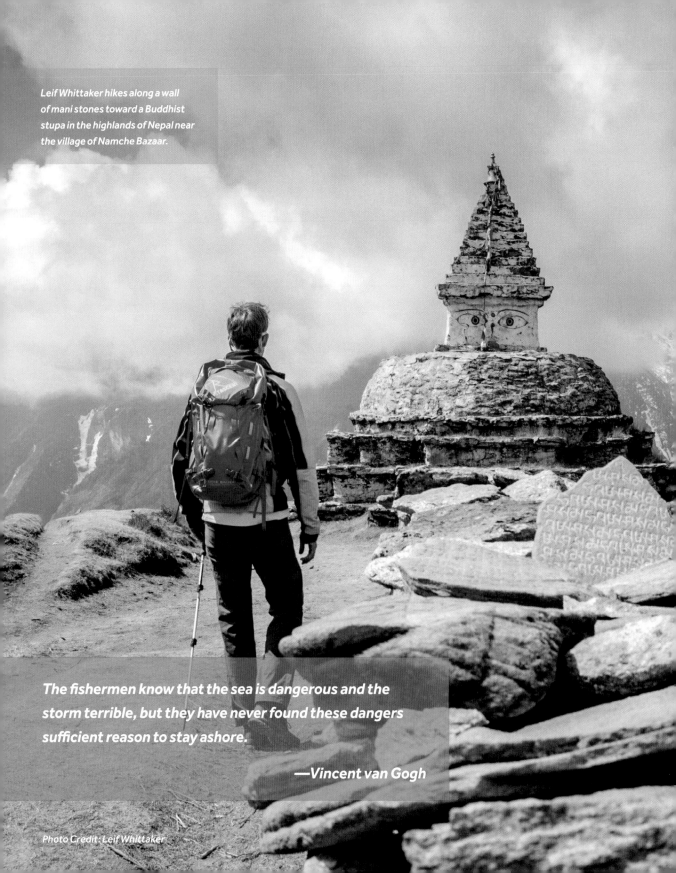

Leif Whittaker hikes along a wall of mani stones toward a Buddhist stupa in the highlands of Nepal near the village of Namche Bazaar.

The fishermen know that the sea is dangerous and the storm terrible, but they have never found these dangers sufficient reason to stay ashore.

—Vincent van Gogh

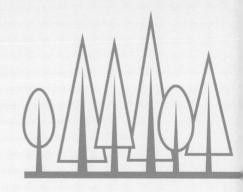

CHAPTER 4
ROUTING OUR WAY BACK TO NATURE

A study by the Environmental Protection Agency found the typical adult spends 93 percent of their time indoors (86 percent in buildings and another 7 percent in vehicles), while the average child is outside for less than thirty minutes a day. As a result, we're becoming nature-phobic, losing even a basic understanding of the world around us and creating biological and psychological problems that didn't exist before the Industrial Revolution. We're also creating convenient lies to explain our housebound existence, such as that being outside in winter causes colds, when in fact concentrations of pollutants are two to five times higher indoors and are often the real cause of our sniffles.[76]

Refamiliarizing ourselves with the outdoors is what we so desperately need. We're not going to learn anything meaningful about nature from books or documentaries; we have to go out and experience all it has to offer for ourselves. This doesn't have to be radical or dramatic, or involve traveling to a hotspot like Yellowstone or Sunset Beach. Rather, just start seeing what's close to your home and exploring it. Maybe it's a bike path by a river, a local lake, or a nature center your kids would enjoy. Just spending a little time outdoors is all you need to change your indoor lifestyle for the better.

The Draw of the Great Outdoors

We may be living our lives indoors—from home to the office to the gym—but we were made for the outdoors, literally. Our bodies need sunlight to set our circadian rhythms and to generate vitamin D. (It's no surprise that vitamin D deficiency has soared in the US in the last twenty years—even when we are outside, we're using sunscreen, which effectively stops the production of vitamin D from sunlight.) And spending time outdoors inherently means spending time moving, whether we're walking or surfing or gardening, and that means that we feel better and are healthier.

Break Out of the Big Fitness Prison

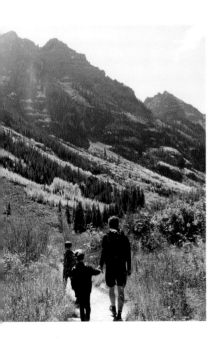

We've been convinced that the only way to "get fit" is to be trained within the confines of a gym, spin studio, group fitness class, and so on. But we conveniently forget that any kind of indoor workout is limited by the equipment, the environment, and the boundaries of physical walls, which in turn limits our development and caps our learning. How do we bust out of this house arrest? Embrace nature, which has no such restrictions.

A big reason that Kai Lenny seems so joyous when he's surfing, stand-up paddleboarding, kitesurfing, or windsurfing is that, while his sponsors compensate him, he still retains the same sense of playful exuberance that attracted him to the water as a knee-high grom. "The ocean is the biggest playground in the world, and it's for free," Kai told me. "No one owns it. You can go out there, and whether you're the poorest or richest person in the world it's going to treat you the exact same. It's the only equal platform on the planet for everybody. Land is just stagnant, still. Water is constant movement and gives us the chance to harness this amazing energy."[77]

Even though Kai is pushing the boundaries in so many sports, the internet-breaking aerial that he pulled off at Jaws in 2016 wasn't an end point for him. Far from it.

> I don't think the trick I did at Peahi was anything special because to me it was just the beginning of where I want to take surfing in the future. Snowboarding was basically born out of surfing. Now it's giving back because I'm looking to surf giant waves as if I was Travis Rice out in Alaska, riding these huge mountains and doing giant tricks. Then you take foilboarding and it's like snowboarding powder. It can give you new opportunities because now you don't have to go surf a crowded break anymore. A crummy wave that you would never have looked at twice becomes something you can surf. Foiling is going to open the world up to more surfers, because it allows us to ride waves that used to be unrideable. I'm trying to build on what Laird [Hamilton], Dave [Kalama], and the Strapped Crew started, and now I see these little kids doing tricks that the pros weren't even trying when I was growing up. Imagine how good they're gonna be in a few years. There are endless possibilities, and surfing will never stop evolving.[78]

One of the keys to lifelong health and fulfillment is to make learning and growth the kind of never-ending, continually evolving process that Kai is talking about. Our opportunities and potential to advance and develop are restricted when we use up all of our active time indoors but unbound when we're outside. When we cultivate an outdoor lifestyle, it becomes effortless to make movement part of our lives, rather than setting aside this little block of time to go to the gym and closing it off from every other part of our day. If you also start to do other things outdoors when the weather permits, like walking to get your newspaper instead of having it delivered, driving to your local park to run sprints instead of cranking up the speed on a treadmill, taking camping vacations, and so on, you soon wonder why you were spending all that time inside. Then you add this to starting a new outdoor sport or picking up an old one (remember that surfboard that's been gathering dust in your garage for the past five years?). And you don't need to wait until you can afford expensive gear like a $600 driver or a $300 tennis racket. Just start playing.

Andy's brother is a good example of someone who did exactly that. When he lived with Andy he had access to a full training gym, kickboxing equipment, and all the other gear Andy has at his house. But when he moved into his own apartment, he had no equipment, no training gear, and no specialist clothes. He just began driving to the nearest ranger station, getting a map, and hiking out into the backcountry. In doing so (tech-free, I might add), he lost a lot of weight and felt his fitness steadily improving. Soon he was ready to take on the 52 Hike Challenge—a movement that calls for people to complete one hike every week for a year—which he completed.

The 52 Hike Challenge website and app are examples of how technology can encourage people to get outside and be more active in nature. They give you tips on how to start hiking, location suggestions based on your skill and experience level, and more. See if your area has a similar online program or app, or ask a park ranger or a friend who's a gung ho hiker. You could also search online for nearby outdoor sports events you might like to try competing in. Exploring different venues, meeting new people, and traversing unfamiliar terrain will encourage you to test your skills, expand your network, and go beyond what you thought you were capable of.

Green Up Your Life

In addition to getting out in nature more, you'd also do well to let more nature in. Andy has found that he's more relaxed since placing potted plants around his office, and these effects aren't merely anecdotal. Houseplants remove up to 87 percent of the volatile organic compounds (VOCs) that get produced in an indoor environment every twenty-four hours and cause everything from minor respiratory issues to more serious health problems like nervous system damage. Adding some greenery can also increase your oxygen intake, as plants release it after taking in and processing carbon dioxide. Plus, the Royal College of Agriculture in England discovered that workers who put plants in their offices improved their attentiveness by 70 percent. (How else do you think we got this book finished?).[79]

The Modern Vampire and Perma-Dusk

Ralph Waldo Emerson once advised his readers to "live in the sunshine, swim the sea, drink the wild air." Most of us don't even get to the sea and wild air parts and are challenged enough just to live a *little* in the sunshine. Vampires avoid sunlight because they die if they're exposed to it. So what's our excuse? Even when we do decide to break our home-work-gym-mall-home cycle of indoor living and dare to venture outside for just a few minutes, we wear sunglasses. As a result, we're living in a state of near-permanent dusk, and our circadian rhythms are the worse for it.

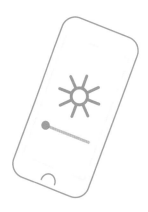

The light that we are exposing ourselves to is harsh and artificial, and it's playing havoc with our eye function. Try turning your phone or tablet to the lowest brightness setting. Then go into a dark room and turn the device on. You'll be amazed by how much light is coming out of that little screen. Consider that most of us actually have our gadgets set to maximum brightness and are staring at them for ten hours or more a day.[80] No wonder "digital eye strain" is a thing now.

Secondhand Nature

In his disturbing dystopian novel *The Circle*, Dave Eggers gives us a withering commentary on people who live vicariously through the social-media posts of others. "You comment on things and that substitutes for doing them. You look at pictures of Nepal, push a smile button, and you think that's the same as going there," Eggers writes. "What would happen if you actually went?" We do this with extreme sports, too, liking or retweeting a video of Jeremy Jones carving his way down an impossibly steep mountainside, Paige Alms escaping from the curl of a giant wave just before it swallows her, or Danny MacAskill doing flips over centuries-old stone walls in the Scottish Highlands. Kai Lenny puts it this way: "It's ridiculous when you see someone just looking at nature on a phone in front of them. It's made-up fun. It's like eating something synthetic versus the real thing, such as a synthetic avocado. Nothing is better than a real avocado."[81]

While we might never reach the level of performance that Kai, Danny, or Paige has obtained, we can at least try to experience more for ourselves and indulge less in what others are doing. This doesn't just encompass sports but everyday activities, too. If you're spending time watching friends' Facebook videos instead of taking your kids to the park to throw a Frisbee or joining them in the driveway to shoot hoops, you need to take stock of your priorities.

To overcome this, try to get more natural light and less of the artificial substitute. During unavoidable screen time, switch your devices to their lowest light settings and use apps like f.lux to dim your displays automatically at certain times of day and night. Next, make an effort to get outdoors at least a couple of times a day, taking your Ray-Bans off unless you're going to be exposed to direct sunlight glaring off snow or water. Make an effort to get your vitamin D through twenty minutes of outdoor time rather than popping a pill. And if you have rooms in your house that naturally get a lot of light, try opening the blinds when you're indoors instead of turning on overhead lights and lamps. Got a deck? Walk back and forth across it when you're on a call rather than plopping down in that recliner or your office chair. Need to meet with a colleague at work? Take a page out of Steve Jobs's book and have a walking meeting to the local coffee shop and back rather than spending another hour in that dreary conference room.

Become a Nature Addict

Earlier we looked at how exercise and technology can combine to become an unhealthy super-addiction. Yet if we switch out the tech component for nature, we can replace the extrinsic rewards that our gadgets provide with the intrinsic rewards of being outside. Sometimes it takes finding an outdoor activity that you enjoy so much, you have to keep coming back to it time and again. A lifestyle sport like surfing calls to people day after day. I'm lucky enough to live in California and so can get out in the ocean year-round, although I admit that I don't surf or paddle nearly often enough.

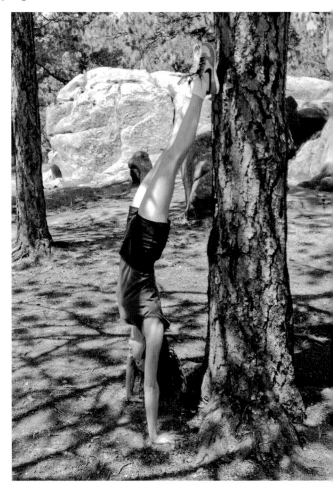

The pull of the mountains is just as strong. In her book *Facing the Extreme*, alpinist Ruth Anne Kocour writes, "Mountaineering is a white-hot imperative—that single interest in life that motivates me in everything else I do. On a mountain, I find that I am able to peel away the camouflage under which all humans hide and experience existence in a pure state—stripped to the bare essentials—life in the raw with its flaws and beating heart exposed for all to see. It is this baring of one's soul that leads to personal awareness and the feeling that one is truly alive."[82]

You don't have to become a surfer or a mountain climber; just find something that captivates you and leads you outside as often as you're able. It might be a solitary pursuit, like snowshoeing, or something you do with friends or a family member, such as hiking every Thursday before work. Once you've found your thing, you won't even have to make a conscious effort to go out and do it—it will just become a part of you. Stepping out into nature shouldn't become yet one more thing you feel obligated to do. Rather, it should be an open invitation that you answer freely in the spirit of conservationist John Muir, who famously wrote, "The mountains are calling, and I must go."

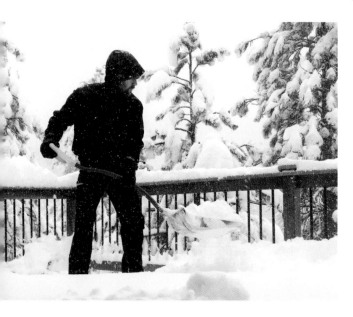

Digital Detox

With our ever-connected lives, we're lacking not just immersion in nature but also time alone and in silence. All three are worth seeking out to re-center ourselves and regain perspective. It's a big world out there, but it's easy to see only our noisy little corner of it. Disconnecting from our devices, spending time outdoors, and seeking out solitude and silence helps us slow down and de-stress, and reminds us that we're part of something bigger than ourselves.

The Value of Feeling Small

One of the things that nature provides and that manmade society cannot replicate is communion with something bigger than us that reminds us of our insignificance. Kai Lenny explained it this way:

The ocean is the greatest teacher ever, and how could you not become part of it at a certain point? Every time I'm in the water I feel like I'm becoming more and more one with it, in my movements, my attitude, and everything else. It has become a part of me as much as I've become a part of it because I'm immersed in it daily. And I'm allowing myself to be. It's this relationship that is as important as any one connection with another human. I probably think about the water more than I think about anything else. Society is a bubble, and every time I go in the water I step outside of it and it's literally the green pasture everyone dreams about. When people talk about heaven on earth, that's how you find it. Right in front of you. You've just gotta look.[83]

Take Your Time

Just as we've been taught to hurry in our jobs, our personal lives, and our workouts, we've also started reducing our experiences in nature to an exercise in time management. Most technology is designed to help us cram more things in by spending less time on each of them, exacerbating the problem. Consider four different ways to see Yellowstone National Park:

1. Flying over in a plane or helicopter
2. Rushing through on a highway at seventy miles an hour
3. Taking a multiday ATV trip
4. Hiking and camping for ten days

Even between options two and three, which are the most similar of the four, it's evident that there would be a significant jump in the quality of your experience if you take an ATV trip. You'd get to go off the beaten path, see waterfalls and rock faces that aren't visible from the main road, and take your time to explore. If you chose option four, you'd remove the noise of a vehicle so that you could immerse your senses more thoroughly, be able to climb trails unsuitable for an ATV, and have that special feeling of exhaustion mixed with deep satisfaction that only comes after walking all day with a pack on your back. The main benefit of option four, though, is that you'd be unhurried and could get in tune with the relaxed rhythms of being in the wilderness. One Finnish study found that it takes eight days to fully de-stress on vacation.[84] So while microdoses of nature are valuable from day to day, it's worthwhile to set aside longer periods to unwind, too.

While it's fun to bring friends or family along, you might want to consider leaving your gadgets behind. There's a reason that more and more resorts are going tech-free: they recognize the value in giving guests a digital detox. Of course, if you're in Yellowstone for ten days, you'll want to take some photos and have a way to contact the outside world if there was an emergency. But turning the trip into an Instagram-fest

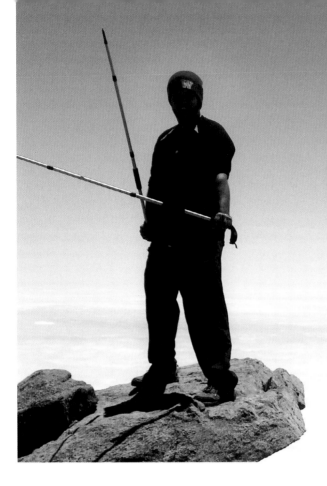

or focusing on your walking pace and mileage the whole time is going to diminish your enjoyment. If you're recording, you're not participating, and if you're capturing, you're not interacting.

To remedy this, you could set a realistic goal, like spending one Saturday or Sunday a month in nature and/or taking a one-week tech-lite or tech-free vacation a year. In addition to setting goals, you could also establish some limits for tech use, particularly when you're outdoors. Maybe try to halve your amount of screen time each day, and use an app like Moment (which allows you to track device usage and set daily limits) to enforce your target if you struggle to stick to your plan. If you're a data geek, you might prefer a tool like BreakFree, which gives you an addiction score based on your gadget use.

Need something a bit more hard-core? Flipd enables you to lock your phone at certain times so there's no chance to cheat. The book *Barbell Buddha*, by Chris Moore, has other ideas for progressions and, as he often puts it, "getting change."

The Gift of Solitude

We're fine to sit at home alone and watch TV or read social-media posts for hours on end, but we're terrified of real solitude and typically avoid any chance of introspection because we're afraid of what we might find. Immersion in the outdoors encourages unfiltered reflection, plus the useful perspective that only comes when pondering something bigger than us. As Aristotle said, "Whoever is delighted in solitude is either a wild beast or a god." When I interviewed Leif Whittaker, the son of the first American to summit Mount Everest, he told me that even as a guide and alpinist, he rarely gets the chance to go off the grid, but when he does, he celebrates it.

"We're so used to being connected that when we're in the wilderness, we feel uncomfortable when our cell phone won't work," Leif said. "But that forces you to disconnect, and if you just go with it, you return refreshed and rejuvenated. It's fun to climb or hike with friends, but there's something about going out alone in nature that replenishes my spirit and heals me."

Unless you're a mountain guide / alpinist / backcountry badass like Leif, you might not have the chance for multiple days of off-the-grid disconnection. So to scale things back to a more obtainable level, make a pledge to spend an hour a week in solitude in some kind of natural environment. If you can't do this in a single block, break it into ten- to twenty-minute daily blocks. You could meditate, read a book, or even listen to music for its own sake, rather just as background noise. Just make sure you're alone and outdoors. So you don't skip such breaks (and, even more so, longer trips), put them on your calendar to make sure they're a priority.

Silence in the Storm

Just as we struggle to come to grips with solitude, I believe we've also lost all ability to be comfortable in silence. That's why many people leave the TV running even when they're not watching it, and why some of us spend hours each day with music blaring from our car radios, at the gym, and through our headphones. As a society, we've made ourselves crave the stimulation of noise and, in doing so, have become allergic to quiet.

Every world religion includes a spiritual discipline that combines quiet and mindfulness—a heightened awareness of ourselves in our environment. There are multiple reasons for this common ground. One is that being still, quiet, and alone offers a daily opportunity to re-center ourselves. If you carve out this time in the morning, it can help focus you on the day ahead. Should you choose nighttime instead, a few minutes of sensory deprivation can clear away hours of anxiety, stress, and worry before you go to bed. But it can be very difficult to find such seclusion in the midst of our hectic world. We're almost always connected and contactable and can usually find multiple excuses to avoid silence and serenity.

This is why we need to seek out nature. Research shows that just looking at landscape photography can lower blood pressure, inflammation, and other stress markers.[85] This effect is amplified when we actually venture outside. Maybe you don't have ready access to unspoiled wilderness, but you don't necessarily need it. One study of people who walked in a busy city found that those whose route took them through green spaces were far more relaxed afterward than the people who stayed surrounded by concrete.[86] And just a little nature goes a long way, with the biological impact lasting for hours following a few minutes of quiet alone time in a natural setting. One tip: leave all your devices at home, because there can be no silence or contemplation when your phone is ringing or your wearable is buzzing.

Finding Freedom

When did we forget how to play? At some point, we began to get all uptight and started to worry about the "right" way to do something, tie ourselves down to measurements of progress and goals, and never stray from the beaten path.

Try setting yourself free from these restrictions and unearth your sense of adventure. Turn off the GPS, immerse yourself in whatever you're doing, and remember what it's like to rely on yourself and your own instincts. Explore. Play. Have fun, and discover things about yourself and the natural world that you never knew.

Never Grow Up

A child doesn't need a rigidly organized workout to have fun and stay healthy while being active. They just get outside and go for it. So why do we adults cling to structure and dogma? We get so hung up on the "right" way to do something that we lose sight of why we fell in love with that sport or activity in the first place. When we get fixated on textbook form or hanging on a certain guru's every word, we're no longer growing but only adhering. This is the exact opposite of the mentality that Bruce Lee had in mind when he said, "Man, the living creature, the creating individual, is always more important than any established style or system."

The self-imposed restrictions of systems don't apply to indoor activities alone but often sadly cross over into our outdoor pursuits. Cyclists get obsessed with maintaining a certain power output, runners on keeping to a mile pace, and alpinists on gaining a certain number of vertical feet. In doing so, they miss out on all the beautiful scenery they're moving across, over, and up. To use a school analogy, we've taken recess away and replaced it with standardized testing. What kid would choose *that*?

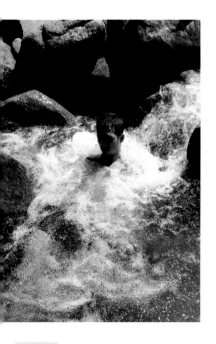

The remedy is to measure less and play more. This is one of the reasons that the "naked" running movement continues to pick up steam. No, the runners aren't dashing around in the nude; they have decided that they no longer want to be tied down by technology. So when a naked runner heads out onto a trail or down a road, the only piece of gear you'll find on them is a water bottle or hydration pack. This way, they can start paying attention to the little things—their feet crunching on crisp leaves, a cool breeze, a magnificent sunset—that were previously obscured by the devices in their pockets, on their wrists, and in their ears. This is how they rediscover movement as play. This is how they reclaim childlike wonder.

Coming back to your natural self can take time. If you go from sitting ten hours a day to standing, you might well develop aches and pains you didn't have before. Or if you go from a sedentary lifestyle to a champion athlete's training plan, you're liable to get hurt real fast. It's better to create and stick to a plan that introduces change gradually. This will allow you to reclaim your physiology without destroying yourself in the process.

Getting Lost, Becoming Found

Whether we're driving to a neighboring town, going on a family road trip, or navigating a trail, many of us long ago ditched our maps for the real-time guidance of GPS. But while this technology seems inherently helpful, it is also changing our brains and killing our built-in sense of direction. The latest research shows that people who learn routes and rely on their own directional instincts are more self-reliant and actually increase the size of their brain's hippocampus by up to 40 percent, as if they were building a muscle through weight lifting. Spatial learning also improves communication between the hippocampus and other regions of the brain and causes synapses to act more rapidly.[87]

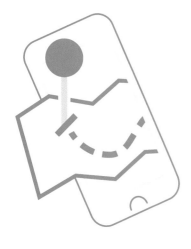

In contrast, always relying on GPS is like giving your brain a test on its sense of direction with the answers already provided. In other words, you don't need to think, reason, or problem-solve. As a result, the brain areas that grow and light up like Times Square on New Year's Eve when we're navigating without satellite assistance stay the same size and remain dull as soon as we ask Siri to take us to the mall.

There's also the issue of spontaneity. If an app or device has outlined your run or ride in advance, you're beholden to starting, following, and ending on this exact path. What if you suddenly get the urge to diverge because you come across a new or partially forgotten road or trail? You should give yourself permission to explore it rather than killing the urge to improvise. The entire concept of rambling—walking through the UK's verdant countryside—is based on walkers having a general sense of where they're going but deciding on their own how best to get there as they traverse fields, cut through forests, and ford streams.

This is not to say that there are no useful applications of GPS. The integration between beacon location tracking and Garmin devices can help rescuers locate someone who has become hopelessly lost in the backcountry, and if you're paddling in unfamiliar open water, having an electronic aid in addition to your own navigational acumen is useful in both sticking to your intended course and getting back to shore safely.

Total Immersion: "You Slip, You Fall, You Die"

In a profile for *Men's Journal*, writer Joseph Hooper outlined the stark reality that free climber Alex Honnold confronts every time he's on a rock face: "No rope, no gear besides rock slippers and a chalk bag, no plan B. You slip, you fall, you die."[88] Most of us would view what Honnold does as crazy, but to him, the kind of total immersion and commitment required to scale thousand-foot walls of granite is what he lives for. And you don't do that kind of living in a sanitized fitness studio.

A key component of Honnold's survival are the instincts he has honed over years of dedicated practice. If he lightly touches a piece of "rotten" rock that feels crumbly, he recognizes that he can't grab on to it without it giving way. Should he look at the sky before an ascent and see a certain type of cloud formation, Honnold knows he has to postpone his climb until the next day so he doesn't get stuck in a thunderstorm. He doesn't need an app or website to tell him these things—his intuition has been finely tuned out of necessity and countless hours spent in the wilderness.

In bouldering, obstacles on rock faces are known as "problems," which is a nice way of implying that the cerebral component is just as important, if not more so, as the physical ability to surmount the challenge. Sometimes these problems are so complex that climbers set up replicas of them in their backyards and spend weeks, months, or even years trying out different resolutions, knowing that one error will have far greater consequences when they're on the actual rock face. This is the kind of simulation Tommy Caldwell did thousands of times in preparation for his and Kevin Jorgeson's boundary-breaking free ascent of Yosemite's Dawn Wall. It took them seven years to feel like they were ready.[89]

And yet for all the prep work, at a certain point, guys like Caldwell, Jorgeson, and Honnold need to just get out there and do their thing. "The thing about suffering is that you don't really need to train to suffer. You just do it. And I think I'm getting better at it. Like, it's feeling more and more mellow," Honnold told Men's Journal. Then there's the issue of actually getting to the wall itself through remote and often treacherous terrain, such as a trip Honnold took in Patagonia. "It's six-hour approaches with a 50-pound backpack, and you're definitely in pain," he said. "It's very unpleasant. But at the same time, I was like, 'This is the most beautiful place on Earth. This is amazing!' It doesn't matter whether it's a good experience or a bad one. Either way you're like, 'Well, I'm just out there having an experience.'"[90]

Yeah, but I'm not going to free solo El Capitan, I hear you saying. Maybe not, but emulating Alex Honnold isn't the point. What I'm trying to convey is our need to be fully present and engaged with something every day, and to have frequent experiences that require us to hone our intuition and problem-solving skills in nature. So find your metaphorical wall, whatever that is, and go climb it.

To retrain your sense of direction, try going off the trail on a short hike and not looking at the signs to get back. No real danger will be present, but you'll probably feel like it the first couple of times until you retune your directional sense. If you've never done it, compete in an individual contest with other people watching, where pride is at stake, like a one-on-one basketball game, a wrestling match, or even an arm wrestle at your local pub. It might feel uncomfortable initially, but such an experience will demand a new level of focus that you can then apply to other areas of your life.

What's Your Quest?

Why is it that fictional stories like *The Lord of the Rings* and real-life ones such as *The Revenant* and *Wild* inspire us?

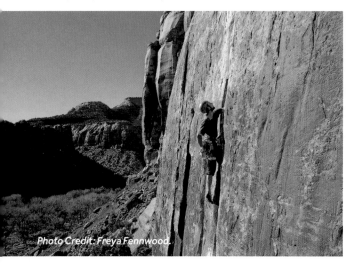

Leif Whittaker climbs **Generic Crack (5.10-)** *in Indian Creek, Utah.*

Photo Credit: Freya Fennwood.

Because they are chronicles of quests in which the heroes encounter suffering and adversity, grow because of it, and finally reach their ultimate goals. Another reason we gravitate toward such tales is that the experiences they portray are very different from those most of us have in our daily lives—they're raw, dangerous, vital.

We were not created to sit in cubicles and traffic jams or wait in Black Friday lines like sheep. Rather, we were made to explore and to conquer. As Helen

Keller wrote, "Life is either a daring adventure or nothing." The difference between most people and pioneers like Conrad Anker, Jimmy Chin, and Sarah Outen is that they've fanned the flame of adventure instead of extinguishing it through a combination of conformity and indoor living. The first step to rediscovering our wild side? Walking out the front door.

Embracing Fear

Fear isn't necessarily a bad thing. It tests us, sharpens our abilities, and shows us what we're truly capable of. It's often when we're afraid that we feel the most alive. But most of the time, we try hard to avoid fear by controlling as much of our environment as we can. It's an understandable impulse, but one that nature doesn't accommodate. It's impossible to control the natural world. So what if we embraced that lack of control instead? What might the fear we face in an uncontrolled situation teach us about ourselves?

You Are Not in Control

Staying indoors all the time furthers the illusion that we can control our environment and minimize, or maybe even eliminate, risk. As Frank Merritt told me when we were brainstorming for this book, "If I'm cold, I'll turn the heat up; if it's too dark in my living room, I'll turn on another light."[91] In-home systems now allow us to do such things with one touch from anywhere.

Such convenience sure is, well, convenient, but it's also reinforcing our need to micromanage every aspect of our world and perpetuating our ability to do so. Helicopter parents are doing the same in trying to create these adversity-free, perfect little worlds to cocoon their kids in. "Then that child grows into an adult who loses it when she has a wrinkle in her shirt and throws a tantrum at Starbucks when her latte is the wrong temperature," Frank said.[92] Technology has furthered our belief that we can control everything. If we're monitoring our bodies round the clock, then we think we have our well-being within our grasp. But if this is true, why are there chronically obese people walking around with wearables?

Fortunately, there is something that offers a reality check and exposes this übercontrol mentality for the lie that it is: nature. No matter how competent and able to shape events we think we are, being outside in an untamed environment reminds us of our insignificance and powerlessness. Laird Hamilton has said that "we're all equal before the wave." If this is the perspective of the world's greatest waterman, how much can the rest of us learn about humility and our inability to bend nature to our will by being out in the water? Or by sitting on top of a mountain peak and watching the sun set above fields of mist? As Lenny Wiersma asked me rhetorically when I was writing this book, "How many pictures of a sunset have been better than any sunset you've actually stood there and experienced?"[93]

If you want to deal with your control issues, commit to doing something once a week that involves being in a situation that's outside your control. Learn to overcome your frustration, to move more freely, and to be open to more possibilities than you could ever imagine when stuck in a gym. You'll find that you can think more creatively and improve your problem-solving skills, as well as spike your awareness.

Scare Yourself Today

We can go through life trying to avoid being scared because society has taught us that fear is negative. But there's something elemental about feeling afraid that isn't all bad. Think about the thrill you got the last time you watched *The Shining* or another horror film, or even a tense drama that provided a few well-timed jump-out-of-your-seat moments. When we confront something that makes us afraid, it forces us to overcome our preconceptions and wrestle with reality in its starkest form. You also have to control your initial reaction—

often fight-or-flight—and problem-solve on the fly to find the best way to deal with the situation in the moment. You don't need to swim with sharks or climb Everest to reap the benefits of being scared. Just being outside in an unfamiliar, uncontrollable situation once in a while will help you master your worries and redefine what you think you're capable of. We supposedly live in the Age of Fear because of our sensationalist press and the hyperbole of social media, but the fears these create and exaggerate in our living rooms—of superbugs, severe weather, politicians who are out to destroy our way of life, and so forth—are not the fears that we need to recognize, embrace, and reckon with when we're out in nature. We need to start minimizing our exposure to the former to overcome the effects of chronic stress and increasing the frequency with which we seek out the latter, because of the lessons that kind of fear teaches us about ourselves, our emotions, and how we can better interact with our living world.

Fear is one of our most primal emotions, and our responses to it are governed by what's known as our "old brain," the part that governs survival instincts and was the first to develop. We engage the fight, flight, or freeze mechanism superficially with the stress we create in our frantic lifestyles, but rarely do we put ourselves in scenarios in which we're exposed to something primal and are forced to moderate our reaction to it. Nor do we seek out activities in which we have to channel all our resources into just making it through. To me, doing so is a part of being fully alive. Kai Lenny agrees: "Exposing yourself to one scare a day is a good thing. It keeps you on your toes, keeps you humble, and keeps your mind open. Put anyone in nature and they go from the top of the food chain to the bottom of it instantly. We've become too elite for nature in our own heads, and that breeds overconfidence that can be self-destructive. Every time you go in the water it teaches you humility, and that's how you survive."[94]

Stayin' Alive

One reason that nature is so restorative is that it forces us to stop worrying about our self-created, first-world problems and our self-actualization wants, and returns our attention to basic survival needs. Kai Lenny offers an example.

I was kitesurfing five miles from my house on Maui and the wind started dying and turning offshore. I was in a position where, okay, I could self-rescue and swim in right where I started, but I decided that I'd just kitesurf down to my house and get a ride back up to my car. So I started going down the coast. About three miles down, the wind began turning more and more offshore. I got blown all the way to the outer reefs, which are at least a mile from land. Then the wind died. The sun had set and it was starting to get dark. Then I noticed there was this shark following me. I had to roll up my twenty-four-meter line and was trying to get my stuff together quickly. Then the wind turned straight offshore again and started blowing me out to sea. The shark was still right there.

My board was too small to prone paddle in on my stomach. I realized I had to swim. So I tacked my board to my kite, which was still inflated but inverted. It was dragging in the water as I tried to swim a mile to shore against the wind. The whole time I was opening my eyes to see if there was anything below me because in most shark attacks it hits you from the bottom. If it went for me I was going to punch it in the nose because this will usually make it wig out and clear off. But the timing is crucial. You have to wait until it's basically on

you. Luckily the shark didn't come for me and I made it back to shore, but it was completely dark and I was wiped.

I guess the moral of the story is just keeping cool under pressure. If at any point you panic, there's a good chance that you're stuck out there. There's no one else that's going to help you. You can't get wrapped up in emotions or what you think other people would tell you to do. You just have to assess the situation, decide to survive, and make it happen. I go into this survival mode that allows me to quickly look at what's happening, anticipate what's next, and make a decision. Because I'm in the water almost every day I can skip a step in that process, and it's like I'm the viewer watching someone else do what's needed. My body just automatically takes over. I think people who are used to being in the mountains or the ocean would have such a higher survival rate if there was an apocalyptic event because these environments make you more aware of your surroundings. We're meant to be instinctual creatures, but we distance ourselves from that because we're living these hollow shells of lives through our screens. You don't have to surf big waves. Just go for a walk in the sand every day or whatever you like to do outside.[95]

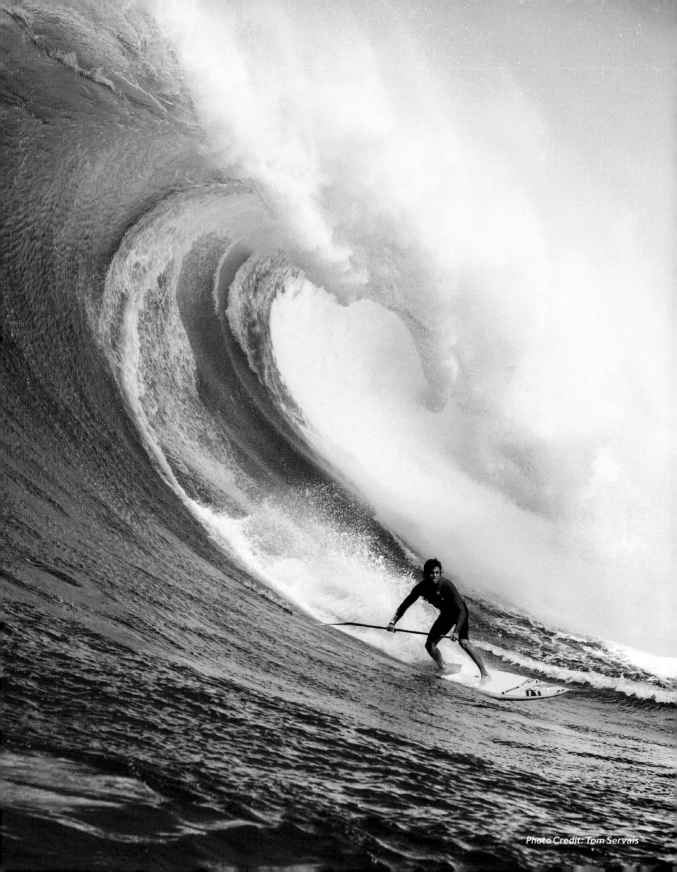

Elemental Healing

We've already mentioned the benefits of being in touch with the elements and not using technology to blunt them. But we'd be remiss to restrict ourselves to the obvious elements of sunlight, wind, and hot and cold. There are substances that are abundant in nature that often go unnoticed but have the power to restore our bodies. Take salt, for example.

"You hear about pro athletes putting sea salt in their baths or swimming in saltwater pools, but why not just go for the real thing in the ocean?" Kai Lenny asked me.

> Sea salt is a healing agent and just one of the beneficial properties we're exposed to when we're swimming, surfing, or paddling. The majority of our planet is made up of water, our bodies are mostly water, and all life came from it.
> Take any grumpy, bummed-out person, put them in the water, and let them swim around for a little bit. Even if they won't admit it, you will notice a physical change in them. You can visually see that their body is a lot more relaxed. If someone is sick or injured and goes in the saltwater every day, I guarantee their chances of getting better shoot through the roof. There's something in the ocean that we can't fully understand, but we can see its effects.[96]

Writer Steven Kotler is living proof of this. He struggled to overcome the ill effects of Lyme disease in his midthirties and his doctors had all but given up. No medicine seemed to work. Steven eventually found his cure from an unlikely source: surfing. He isn't sure what the mechanism for his recovery was, but the fact remains that for him and many others who've been failed by traditional therapies, nature really is the best healer. (See chapter 9 for Steven's back-to-nature tips). Some of us get a similar, if less dramatic, restorative effect from the cold, crisp mountain air, the warm, ambient blanket of the sand dunes, the gigantic mysticism of uncut tundra, or the serenity of a stream running gently through an uninhabited meadow.

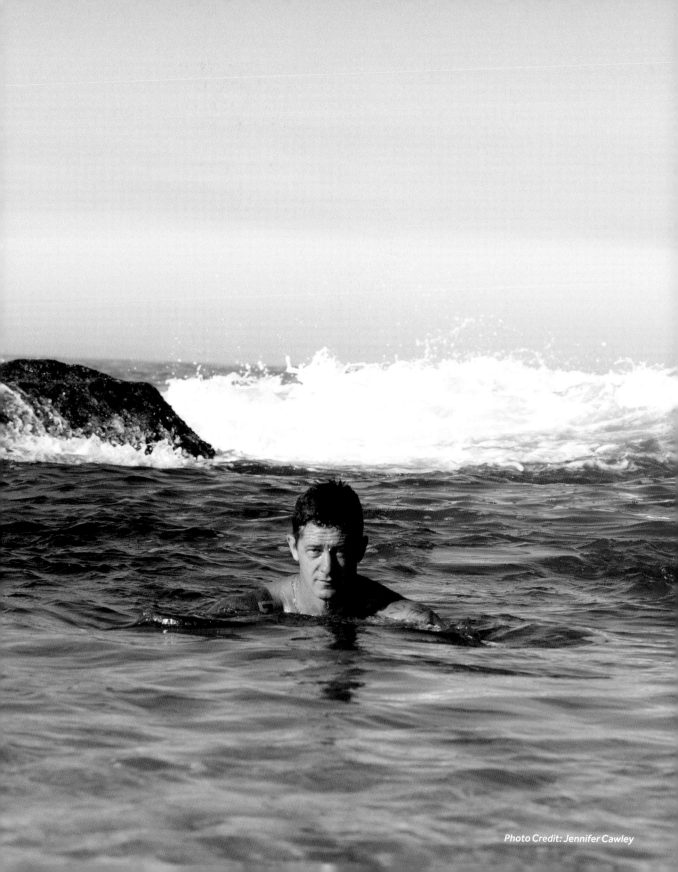

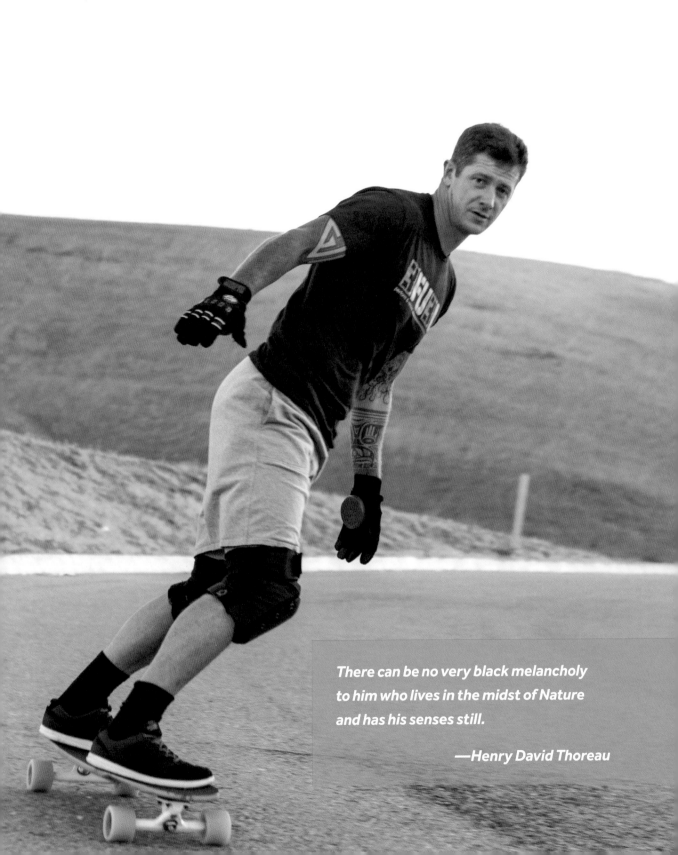

*There can be no very black melancholy
to him who lives in the midst of Nature
and has his senses still.*

—Henry David Thoreau

CHAPTER 5
USING SENSES, NOT SENSORS

To be fully engaged with the world around us, we need to be fully conscious of it and ourselves. And yet, as Larry Rosen puts it in his book *iDisorder,* from the moment we first check our phones in the morning we're being "pulled into a world of button clicks, finger swipes and glowing screens" from which some of rarely emerge.[97] This leads to our dulling our perceptions and senses and continually upping our reliance on technological sensors—which mandate the route we're traveling, control the temperature of our cars and homes, tell us what appointment we've got to go to next—to guide our decisions and actions.

In terms of our health and performance, we're also delegating more and more to our devices. Want to know if you're going too fast or too slow? Listen to the coach in your ear. Not sure if you're adequately hydrated? Wait for your smart water bottle to tell you when to drink. Can't decide if you're just a bit sore or too fatigued to train? Let your heart rate monitor make the call. Let's look at just how far the senses versus sensors seesaw has tipped toward technology, and what you can do about it.

Engineering Discomfort and Manufacturing Suffering

As a society, do we care about anything as much as being comfortable? From multizone heating and cooling at home and work to dual-zone climate control and cold-weather packages in our cars, we go out of our way to never feel extremes of temperature or weather. As a result, we've suppressed our innate regulation ability, which kept ancient tribes alive as they migrated across searing deserts and frozen tundra.

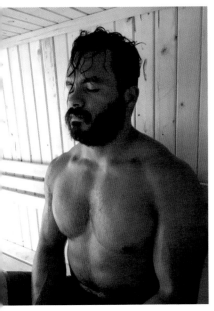

To counter the comfort we've engineered in so many aspects of our cushy, abundant lives, we feel the need to come up with artificial experiences that expose us to the kind of extremes that help us not only self-regulate temperature but also to feel. This is why I join my friends and colleagues Laird Hamilton, Gabby Reece, and Wim Hof in dunking myself in an ice bath and sweating out in a dry sauna three times a week, and why I take freezing showers every other day. It's also the reason we hurl ourselves into icy pools during obstacle races and test our endurance in extreme environments, such as running across Death Valley in the Badwater Ultramarathon or, in Wim's case, completing marathons across the Arctic Circle in nothing more than a pair of shorts.

You don't need to go to such lengths. But it'd be worthwhile to get uncomfortable more often and rely on technology less as you're doing so. Instead of setting the air in your car to

Photo Credit: Bryan Diaz

63 degrees, roll down the windows and let some fresh air in. Go for a run in the heat of the day sometimes instead of in the cool of the early morning—and do it tech free. Test out that plunge pool that nobody uses at your health club. By giving our bodies and brains stimuli outside of the narrow range of comfort we've created, we can help reawaken everyday sensation and prepare our bodies to self-regulate when we have to face the extremes—even if that's just shoveling the driveway when it's 20 degrees outside or doing that charity bike ride with our kids in the middle of an August heat wave.

Another benefit to the heat/ice practice is that it can't be done when hooked up to a device. Constant connection to our tech toys makes it more difficult than ever to set aside personal time in which we're doing restorative activities—like meditating or praying, breathing, or even just taking a soak—without monitoring. We need to think more deeply about the consequences of this tethering, and make more of an effort to create moments of introspection in which we're not focused on an external object but on our inner selves.

Avalanche!

One of the instincts that Laird Hamilton has honed over the years is his ability to sense danger before it manifests itself and to take corrective action. When you're dealing with multistory waves, failure to do so can be fatal. Laird has found that this highly sensitive built-in early-warning system also works when he trades water for snow.

"I was in Alaska snowboarding with a friend in an area known for its frequent avalanches," Laird said. "He was about to start another run and I felt like something was off. I knew something bad was about to happen, so I grabbed his jacket and pulled him back to stop him. Right after I did that, this wall of snow blasted right through where he would've been. It would've taken him out."[98]

Paying Attention to Your Body

We're so used to living in our heads—thinking about a problem at work, what we need from the store, or what's going to happen if we can't complete this next rep—that we forget to pay attention to what our body is telling us. It's sending us messages all the time about how it's doing and what's going on around us. Learning to listen to this biofeedback is an essential part of reconnecting to ourselves and our practice.

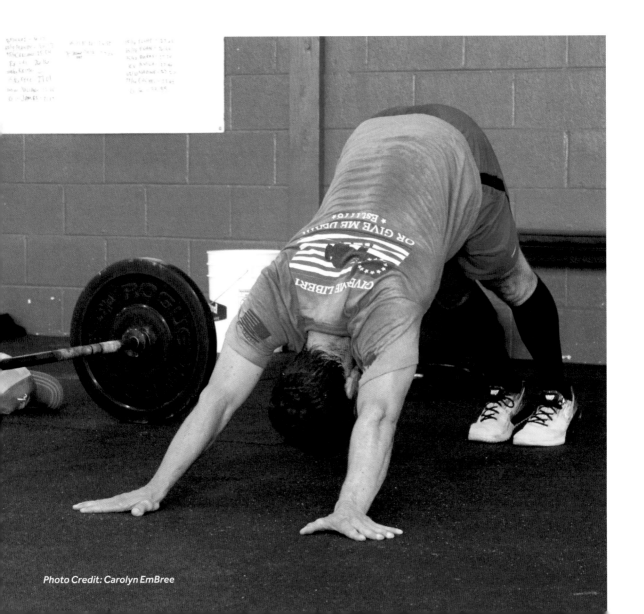

Photo Credit: Carolyn EmBree

When You Break

An important step in improving your self-awareness is to see how you feel when your breathing pattern is unsustainable or when your position breaks, and to recognize whether what you do next is helping or hurting you. Something I see frequently is that when endurance athletes cross their lactate threshold, they gasp, yawn, or take a double breath to try to take more oxygen in. Do they know how it feels to cross that line, and do they recognize how they're changing their breathing to compensate as they do so? If they've checked both those boxes, do they also understand how to implement a better breathing strategy and how this will help their performance?

Technology can help here by providing instant feedback while you're still exercising, in two ways. First, if I were measuring your oxygen saturation, I'd know when you were about to hit an energy system threshold. Second, a video of you at this point would show that you took a quick double breath, yawned, or lapsed into an irregular breathing pattern that's different from the one you started the session with. Once you recognize what you're doing and when, it's easier to connect sensation ("I feel short of breath...") to physiology ("...when I cross my lactate threshold...") to an action ("...so I take a double breath and my breathing pattern falls apart...") and finally, to a consequence ("...and my final split time is terrible").

Then I could introduce the solution so you could explain it to me ("I need to start out with a more sustainable breathing pattern" or "I need to switch to take a double breath but then return to my breathing cycle"). Once you've made the connections among what's happening, why, what you're doing about it, and how you can do better, then you've developed the self-awareness to problem-solve independently.

We can sometimes panic when our body freaks out. Frank Merritt and Brandon Rager, who played in the NFL, see this in their work with football teams. A sense of powerlessness over our own bodies is especially acute when we experience problems with our breath, because breathing is so essential. So if a football player is short of oxygen because he is breathing poorly or his cardiovascular training has been lacking, he's going to start taking short, staccato breaths. These signal his body to go even deeper into sympathetic high alert, which further disrupts his oxygen intake. It's a vicious cycle. But if we can intervene and use technology as a teaching aid that connects his issue (being short of breath) to what his body is struggling with (low oxygen levels) and then to a solution (controlled diaphragm breaths for now, a cardiovascular training program for later), the panic goes away.

Test Your Senses

To fully recognize how thrown-off your senses likely are from your lack of attentiveness to them, you could try these four easy sensory experiments.

Smelling: Try to go a week without exposing yourself to any artificial scents off any kind. This means giving cologne, detergents, and air fresheners the heave-ho. At the same time, make an effort to be more aware of natural scents. Try rubbing herbs like rosemary or sage between your fingers. If you go for a run on a winter day, home in on the smell of a wood-burning fire. Cook a curry dish and pay attention to the scent of each spice.

Tasting: Make an effort to eliminate as much sugar from your diet as you can. That means not sweetening your coffee, ditching desserts, and drinking green tea with nothing added, for example. After a few days, add in only natural sugars, like those found in fruit and honey. See how these taste compared to artificial sweeteners you may have used before, and how your tolerance for sweetness has changed. You could also do the same with added salt.

Hearing: Start listening to music and your TV at the lowest possible volume. This might mean gradually lowering the output over a week. At the end of the experiment, I bet you'll feel like a lot of things around you—the blaring of a sports game at a restaurant, your buddy's car stereo, and so on— seem far too loud.

Seeing: Commit to setting aside your sunglasses for a week (unless this would dangerously compromise your safety at a certain time of day, such as if the sun is in your eyes when you're driving back from work). By the end of the week, you'll probably find you're no longer oversensitive to sunlight and you notice more details in your surroundings than ever before.

Recalibrating Your Zoom Lens

Our eyes' ideal focal point is twenty feet in front of us, yet we sit for hours a day with screens a few inches from our faces. Because we spend little to no time outdoors in random, chaotic environments that require us to constantly toggle between what's in the foreground, in the distance, and every point in between, our mid- and long-range vision is starting to deteriorate. We're also unlearning how to use our peripheral vision because instead of noticing a deer leaping over a log or a waterfall cascading down a cliff face, our attention is fixed on what's right in front of us.

When she started working with England's rugby team, vision expert Sherylle Calder told *The Telegraph* that technology was hurting players' skills by negatively impacting their vision:

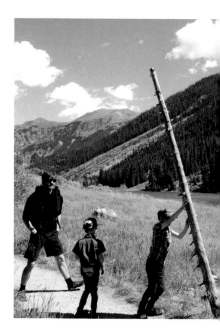

> In the modern world, the ability of players to have good awareness is deteriorating by the nature of mobile phones. . . . We have seen in the last five or six years, when we assess elite players in different sports, that there is a decline in skill levels. When you look at your phone, you are losing awareness, because you're in here [the screen] all the time. There are no eye movements. Everything is pretty static. We are losing the ability to communicate well. . . . We develop skills by climbing trees, walking on walls and falling off and learning all those

visual motor skills, which people aren't doing any more. Young kids spend a lot of time on mobile phones, so those instinctive natural skills are disappearing. If you don't see something, you can't make a decision.[99]

The cure for this is a simple one. When you've been staring at a screen for twenty minutes, find an object in the middle distance and focus your attention on it for at least twenty seconds. Then focus on something that's even farther away (yes, if you work in an office with no windows, you'll need to find one or go outside). To further improve your vision, make an effort to get out in nature at least once a day, even if that's just a city park. And while you're in this setting, make a conscious effort to avoid checking your phone or wearables and notice details about what's going on around you—a squirrel scurrying up a tree, a bird taking flight, grass rustling in the wind.

Can You Hear Me Now?

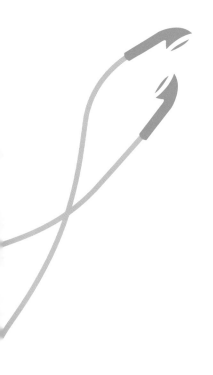

When I was developing the Power Speed Endurance program, I trained hard for the grueling Western States Endurance Run—one hundred miles through the desert—and usually relied on music to help get me through. Since the race is so tough, I figured I should put in my headphones and get some music pumping around fifteen miles into the race itself. But for the next two hours, what I thought would help me actually became a massive hindrance. Because I had my tunes wired in, I tuned out what I was doing with my body, so mechanical errors started to creep in. I also started to make mistakes in how I dealt with the trail itself, which, when you're miles from anywhere, can quickly become a big problem.

So when I got to the next aid station, I threw my iPod and headphones to one of my crew members, got back to focusing on myself and my surroundings, and finished the race. From that point on, I never again used music to help me get through a race or training session. One of my friends, Josh

Everett, once said that if you need music to motivate you to do something, you should find something else to do, and he's right.

That being said, I haven't thrown my headphones in the trash. If I'm running, cycling, surfing, or doing something else outside, I'll just listen to the sounds of nature. But if I'm stuck indoors, I've found the brain.fm app to be very helpful. It generates ambient noise tailored to work, meditation, and various other activities. Rather than making me become semiconscious, as listening to music does, it actually heightens my awareness and engagement with the task at hand. Anytime you can use technology to improve your connection to yourself and your surroundings, do it.

The Equipment Compromise

The equipment we rely on every time we train can feel indispensable. But the truth is, sometimes it's not only unhelpful but actually harmful. Using advanced gear too much or the wrong kind of equipment can end up compromising our technique and lead to injury. It also doesn't prepare us for performing without it, as we may need to in nature or in competition. And finally, total reliance on technology doesn't account for changes in conditions that should influence how we plan and assess our training when the numbers don't tell the full story.

Born to Run Was Right

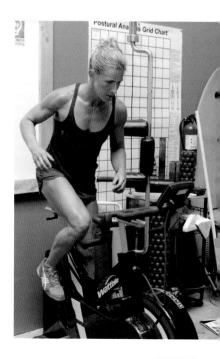

After Chris McDougall released his book *Born to Run* in 2009, thousands of runners realized that overly cushioned shoes were doing them more harm than good, and manufacturers responded to their demands for more flexible, minimal footwear. Soon enough, almost every one of them had low- or zero-drop offerings in their product lineups, while Vibram could barely keep up with demand for its separated-toe, socklike FiveFingers shoe.

McDougall was right on point in calling out the false impression that a piece of technology can massively improve your performance. Yet despite his warnings to slowly transition from overly cushioned, inflexible shoes to minimal models and then to zero-drop ones—all while keeping mileage low—many people ignored this advice and tried to quit their fat-soled shoes cold turkey. This led to an orthopedic disaster. I had people showing up to my seminars who were just trashed and couldn't understand why. They'd tell me things like, "I don't get it…I thought my feet would be healthier if I went barefoot."

Once I dug a little deeper into their stories, I found that not only had they gone from a ten-millimeter or greater heel-to-toe differential to zero drop in one fell swoop, but they'd also kept the same program as they had before they made the switch. Plus, their pampered feet had become weak while cruising around on a couple of inches of midsole foam or air and needed both mobilizing and strengthening through a gradual transition to the way nature intended their feet to function. Yet they didn't know this or glossed over the advice that McDougall and others tried to give, with dire results.

In the wake of a lawsuit against Vibram, all those foot injuries, and other signs that the tide was turning against running barefoot and in minimal shoes, the main manufacturers did what they often do and swung the technology pendulum hard in the other direction. Several new start-ups also entered the market, touting the benefits of their ultrathick, übercushioned soles, which would supposedly right all the podiatry wrongs. Suddenly, shoes were even fatter and less flexible than they'd been before *Born to Run* and the revolution that it birthed. Even those shoemakers who had seemed fully committed to minimalist running began reintroducing arch supports and increasing the drop of their models. While those who had steadily transitioned to barefoot or zero-drop running protested, the mass market embraced the bulky cushioning that was suddenly fashionable again.

It wasn't just the midsoles that got bigger—so did the claims that the shoe companies started making. Now they promised not only to protect your feet from impact but also to track your stride length, cadence, and speed with embedded sensors connected to an app or wearable. Add spongy cushioning to quantification and you get a double dose of desensitization and distraction. What many people don't acknowledge is that all that air under their feet is buffering poor mechanics like overstriding and heel striking, while our shoes' sensors reward us for the faster times that might result. So we're creating bad habits and then positively reinforcing them. It's not until we get injured that we realize something's amiss.

This is why if we're going to reawaken our senses, we've got to stop or minimize our use of all technology that puts a barrier between us and our environment, whether that's two-inch midsoles or anything else. Instead, we should carefully use stripped-down equipment—like minimally cushioned shoes—to improve the feedback of the ground beneath our feet. When we feel that we're overstriding or committing another positional error, we can then focus on the skill element of running to improve our form before we even think about improving our split or lap times.

Losing the Equipment (Dis)advantage

I've been cycling for more than three decades and have clipped into my pedals for as long as I can remember. But one day last year, I was catching up with my friend Jessi Stensland, who's an internationally renowned triathlete. Jessi told me that after taking time off in Costa Rica, she realized how much ankle and foot function she'd been missing. On her trip, she imitated the locals and got down in a deep, butt-to-heels squat every day when playing with kids, sitting around a campfire, and more. At first this was difficult because of her limited ankle mobility. This got her thinking about what had compromised her natural capability. A culprit soon emerged: cycling shoes that kept her foot in a rigid position for the hundreds of training miles she put in each month.

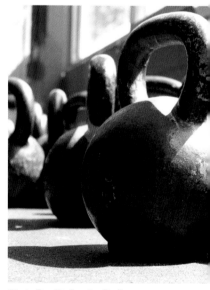

Photo Credit: Carolyn EmBree

Jessi's story inspired me to reexamine my own cycling. Why exactly was I clipping in? Well, there's the fact that pretty much every serious cyclist does it, and the accepted wisdom that doing so allows you to generate more power. But at what cost? So I decided to go back to basics and stop using cycling shoes and clips. It felt weird at first, but I soon recognized that my mechanics were a lot better, as was my positioning on my bike. Yes, I sacrificed a bit of power to begin with, but I soon refined my technique to compensate. As a result, I became more efficient, which enabled me to get that clipped-in speed back.

Are you relying on a piece of equipment in a similar way? Maybe it's a paddle with a huge blade that enables you to generate a lot of power with little thought for stroke technique. Or some fat-soled shoes that allow you to heel strike to your heart's content. Perhaps it's a weight belt you use when you squat in the belief that it will keep your lower back safe when you're packing on all those plates, without realizing that it can encourage you to overestimate your ability and disengage your core, which naturally stabilizes your spine. Take a look at your gear and identify something that's providing a benefit, but at a cost. Then try doing without it for a while and see what you learn about how you can improve your mechanics. Chances are it will take a little discovery and a few setbacks to find your new groove. But you'll be better off in the long run (or ride).

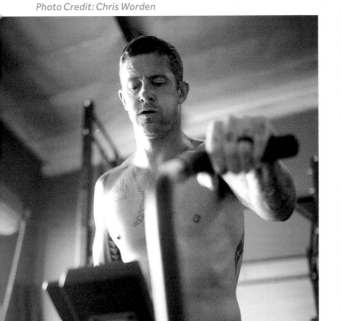

Photo Credit: Chris Worden

Braced for Impact

Another crutch that athletes are overdependent on is braces and supports. This is perhaps most prevalent in basketball, where players who've frequently rolled their ankles not only tape them before games but also strap into braces so tight that they'd make a corset-wearing *Downton Abbey* star feel restricted. The theory here is that if you limit the range of motion at the ankle, you're less likely to turn it when stepping on another player's shoe or landing awkwardly after a layup. But the problem is that the foot-ankle complex becomes weak after a sprain, and it will never regain its integrity or mobility if the player is binding the ankle tightly. Also, the ankle doesn't function in isolation but in a system with the knee and hip. When you land from a jump, your body needs to absorb massive forces, and it naturally does so by flexing simultaneously at the ankle, knee, and hip. But when you block one part of this sequence by bracing the ankle (or, indeed, the knee), you change the movement pattern. If there's a positional error at the bottom of the chain, the body has to make a correction higher up to maintain stability.

Unfortunately for the brace-bound player, such a compensation is often made at the knee. So when the athlete takes a misstep or has an off-balance landing, the ankle might well be protected, but the knee takes the brunt of the twisting force and collapses inward. With some players who've used braces for years, you can see this even occurs to some degree every time they jump—which could happen hundreds of times in each game. As a result, the connective tissues of the knee are placed under excessive strain, and it's often the anterior cruciate ligament (ACL) that gives out first. So you're just trading one issue—a sprained ankle—for another—a blown ACL.

If you suffer frequent ankle sprains, a better approach is to work with a physical therapist on regaining your proprioception—awareness of your limbs' position and posture—after an injury. You should also do a minimum of ten minutes of daily mobility work, as well as improving reactive balance and your single-leg strength with hops, bounds, step-ups, pistol squats, and lunges. In addition, you can work on landing mechanics, lateral movement, and eccentric strength (that is, strength as a muscle is lengthening under load). This will reduce the chance of reinjury and help your ankle function as it should. In addition, you'll avoid the risk of knee damage that those clunky braces exposed you to. You might decide to wear a brace in the first few games after returning from the injury, but you should avoid doing so in practice and try to go brace-free in competition as soon as possible.

Train Like You Compete

Lenny Wiersma has seen that swimmers who most closely replicate race conditions in training often fare better than those who rely on metrics and measurements to guide their training but don't have access to their technology during competition.

"Relying on technology is dangerous because it can limit a person from going from the cognitive stage to the autonomous stage," Lenny said. "If they've been told by this external device in training how they should pace themselves the whole time and then go into a competition, they can fail to recognize that it's completely different. Now they have a human who they're competing against and it's a chess game. An athlete needs to be able to feel and make adjustments."[100]

For surfers like Kai Lenny, the only thing they can rely on when a winter storm rolls in is themselves: "The reality is that you can get stuck when you use technology," Kai said. "Once the waves come, we ditch all that junk. It's just us and the board, and it becomes instinctual, with our experience meshing with what's happening in the now, versus what the outcome should be."[101]

The point here is that if you can't perform at a high level without technology, you've been fooling yourself and don't really have the ability. I'm not saying that using technology is cheating, but we can't look at, say, a new record for climbing Everest in the same way if the climber used oxygen and other technology that the former record holder did not. The truest test of your skill is how well you can accomplish a task when it counts, with the least amount of tech.

Consider the Conditions

Another factor that can change performance is the conditions in which you're training or competing. Sprinters are rarely going to run as fast into a headwind as they would if the wind was still. When there's a tailwind at a track-and-field meet, the maximum for new records to be set is two meters per second. If you're cycling on a ninety-five-degree day in July, your time for a certain ride (not to mention the exertion during and fatigue after, calorie expenditure, and hydration level) might well be different than if you raced the same course when it's twenty degrees in February.

The trouble is that technology rarely takes varying conditions into account. My wife, Erin, gave an example of how this can be misleading.

> If I'm out rowing on a flat day, it's going to take less effort to get to and maintain a certain pace than it would if there was cross-chop or if I was rowing upwind in the ocean instead of on a calm lake. But a monitor wouldn't know what the water or weather was doing, so it might show a slow speed despite all the energy it took to reach that. This is why you need to be able to adjust in the moment and be aware of your exertion level, outside of what the numbers say. It doesn't matter if your device tells you that it was an easy session if you know it was hard. And that can change by how you feel on a certain day, not just because of the environment.[102]

Energy Is Everything

Each winter I spend a few weeks in Hawaii. It's a tradition I started a long time ago, when I was a competitive runner who wanted to get some quality training in and relished the challenge of surfing some of the islands' big winter swells. Over the years, I've backed off the running a bit, kept the surfing, and tried to add a couple of new activities each year, from mountain biking volcanoes to getting my butt kicked by some buddies who also happen to be jiujitsu world champions.

One of the most meaningful experiences I've had in Hawaii occurred in November 2016, when I decided to go out snorkeling with a group of friends, including CrossFit Games competitor Matt Chan (who, by the way, is terrified of open water but a good enough sport to indulge me and push himself past his fear). We were soon joined by some unexpected gatecrashers: about twelve or fifteen sharks, who swam around and underneath us for twenty or thirty minutes. Matt, who is one of the toughest guys I know, started freaking out, and for good reason. Any one of these apex predators could've decided to take a bite out of us at any time. But as I tried to stay open to what was happening and attempted to talk Matt down, I noticed that the sharks did not bring an attitude of intimidation or aggression to our encounter, despite obviously having the upper hand (or fin, if you will). Instead, they seemed to wait to see how we were acting. I find that it's the same around my dogs. They're not going to bite you and will stop barking if you're respectful and behave yourself.

How you project yourself also profoundly impacts how you interact with other people, who make instinctual judgments about your mood and energy from posture, gestures, tone of voice, and facial expressions. And in fact, research shows that the old adage "Attitude follows action" has validity on a biological level, as what we do and how we do it can greatly impact both our own emotions and those of other people. If we can make more of an effort to do things openly and enthusiastically and try to assimilate and learn at all times, we'll get a lot more out of each day because our physiology will reflect our positive psychology and we won't have to waste energy combating a negative or inhibited mind-set. And we don't need an app to prompt or measure such an attitude.

My good friend and former professional volleyball player Gabby Reece takes a very deliberate, proactive approach to

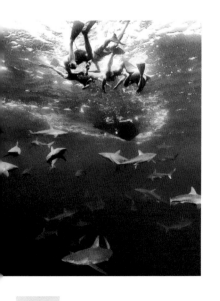

her own attitude and how she impacts those around her. She's committed to "going first" in smiling at people, starting a conversation, and greeting others, recognizing that she can be the one to set the tone of every interaction. Try to emulate her and go first with each person you encounter today, from your loved ones to friends to strangers. Also, learn to control your reactions to negative events, like disagreeing with a colleague, getting cut off in traffic, or receiving the wrong order at a restaurant. If you can do both of these things, you'll better manage your energy and have a more optimistic outlook that leaves a positive mark on those around you.

Going by the Numbers

As important as it is to listen to what our senses are telling us, hard numbers can be helpful, too, whether they come from a device or our own two fingers. Knowing just what our heart rate and oxygen saturation is at a certain point in training can be invaluable. It can even teach us how to slow our heart rate at will.

Fine-Tuning Your Decision-Making

Though it's possible to select activities, decide on intensity and volume, and choose when you need more rest and recovery just based on your feelings in the moment, this has its risks. If you decided, say, that you would not train on days when you felt worn down or burned out, some of those rest days might be legitimate and you'd benefit from the layoff. But because you've given yourself permission to chill out whenever you feel the need, it suddenly becomes easier to write off activity days on which you might be physiologically fine to push yourself hard. The mind has a naughty way of tricking us out of anything that it perceives requires effort. Similarly, you might assume that you're pushing yourself hard on days that are meant to involve a hard effort, but over time your grasp on that can start to slip.

So while I'm not going to contradict myself and say that you always need to use technology to monitor your effort or recovery, it can be useful to fire up a pacing app or use a heart rate monitor once in a while to recalibrate yourself. If you see that your splits are indeed fast during an interval workout, then you'll know that your appraisal of such sessions is right on and you don't need to change a thing. However, if your times are far below what you'd expect, then you'll know you need to dial up the intensity. In that case, try getting to the output level that you want and be conscious of your breathing, heart rate, and energy expenditure when you reach it. Then the next time you do a similar session, you can do it without the aid of technology, using your newly attuned perception as your guide instead.

The same principle can be applied to resting heart rate. If you take your pulse when you get up each morning for a week and see that on a morning that you were feeling wiped, your rate was ten beats higher than on the other days, then you'll have confirmed that your instinct not to train that day was correct. But if the value on that day is similar to the others that week, then perhaps you were trying to con yourself out of hopping on your bike.

Time to Take Your Pulse

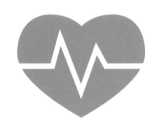

Another way to measure heart rate is with a pulse oximeter, a relatively inexpensive piece of equipment that also lets you look at oxygen saturation. I've used various models over the years, both for myself and my athletes. But one day I started to question how well they actually worked. So I booked time in a lab like Andy's and went there with twenty athletes and several different types of oximeters. The exercise scientists monitored the athletes' pulse rates with professional-grade equipment while we also monitored them with the commercial-grade oximeters. For the first experiment, we had them do five minutes of hyperventilation breathing using the Wim Hof Method. The lab equipment showed oxygen saturation of 98 percent or above. But all the commercially available oximeters registered levels below 90 percent. Conclusion: the oximeters were inaccurate.

Next we looked at pulse rates following intense exercise intervals with several minutes of deep, controlled, relaxing breathing that's meant to send the body from a sympathetic stress state (fight or flight) into a parasympathetic recovery (rest and digest) one. The lab equipment showed that all the athletes' pulses dipped to 100 bpm or below. However, the oximeters registered pulse rates of around 120 bpm, with some even higher. I guess using cheap oximeters isn't the best idea.

Instead, you can take your own pulse using nothing more than two fingers. I press these to the carotid artery on the side of my neck, in the hollow next to my windpipe, and count how many times my heart beats in ten seconds. Then I multiply this by six to get my bpm. You can also take your pulse at your wrist: place two fingers just below your thumb, over your radial artery.

If you're curious about the relationship between oxygen saturation, heart rate, and metabolic pathways (i.e., the ways your body produces fuel from food), you can do a twelve-minute metabolic test that increases the intensity of rowing, cycling, or running every minute; the goal is to reach your max heart rate in the final sixty seconds. With well-conditioned athletes, we usually see an even jump of two, three, or four beats every minute. If someone's pulse jumps by a lot more—say eight or ten beats each minute—we know that they're crossing a threshold and changing the metabolic system they're using, such as transitioning from primarily using glucose and glycogen as fuel to utilizing fat.

The key element here is connecting what's going on with the heart rate and the metabolic pathway with the athlete's sensation. I'll stand beside them and ask what they're feeling. Often they'll say, "My body feels like it's burning" or "I'm out of breath." This is a clear indicator that their heart rate just spiked and that they're also crossing a metabolic threshold. I then explain the correlation to them after the test, so they know what physical sensations to look for next time they're out on a run or bike ride. They can also utilize this self-knowledge to work at a certain intensity so they can improve their ability to sustain power at a certain level. And because they now know what it feels like to reach their max heart rate, they won't need tech to tell them.

Playing the Game

In addition to working with some of the biggest stars in the Olympic swimming pool, Lenny Wiersma also coaches swimmers at UCLA and junior athletes. He has found that he can use heart rate variability technology to help people control their nerves before competition. "I help my athletes learn how to control their physiology by using certain relaxation and breathing techniques," he said.

> First they learn things that they can do without external cues, and then they use the visual feedback to help guide them to do it the right way. And then they do it again without the visual feedback. That way they can access it before competition without needing the technology. They're now able to replicate those breathing and relaxation techniques in this otherwise extremely stressful environment, and it gives them control. It keeps their conscious attention on the present, instead of worrying about their race. We also use a display that starts off with blocks of black and white, but as your heart rate changes, it morphs into other colors. The kids like that because it's like a video game, but one they can control with their pulse by controlling their breathing.[103]

So if you're considering buying a pulse oximeter, heart rate variability monitor, or any other device, consider how you plan to use it to enhance your discovery and consciousness. Don't just do as the instructions say and plug in your age, weight, gender, and so on and go through the motions, because you won't learn anything.

Virtual Reality

We've talked a lot about reconnecting with the physical world—with nature, our bodies and senses, and our environment—and how technology can get in the way of that. But one emerging technology promises to take us further than ever from the real world: virtual reality. That's not necessarily a bad thing if it's used discerningly, but it's worth considering when and how virtual reality may have a place in physical activity.

Is This the Real Life?

Some exercise bikes already enable their riders to join virtual pelotons as they compete in the stages of famous races like the Tour de France. In the next couple of years, such technology will take a giant step forward as gym goers put on virtual-reality headsets and immerse themselves more deeply in detailed terrain. Yet as realistic as such an experience might seem, it's still going to be devoid of actual life. Users will not feel wind blowing in their face or the sun on their back, nor will they have to overcome issues like a slipped chain or the interference of a spectator. Even VR "enhanced" indoor cycling will still be just that—indoor cycling. There's also the point that some of the bikes offering race-related courses are so expensive that for the same price you could actually buy a plane ticket, book a hotel in France for a few weeks, and check out the Tour de France stages for yourself.

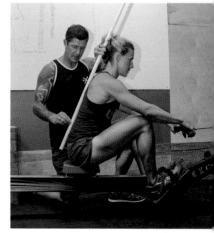

Brian using simple tools like a plastic pipe and a rope to help an athlete understand proper body position and mechanics during the rowing exercise.

Now, if you're kept off the roads by a harsh winter, VR indoor cycling might well suffice as a temporary substitute for the real thing, but if at all possible, the wannabe rider should actually get out, visit some of the courses they want to ride, and try them. Or, if the peaks of the Pyrenees are out of reach, experimenting on different training routes closer to

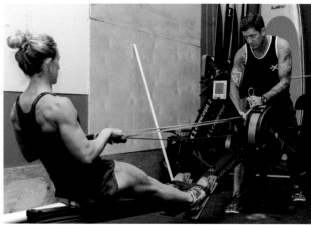

The athlete is then asked to reproduce the position without the tool and maintain proper form as intensity and fatigue increase.

home with friends or entering new races would provide a fresh challenge. For those who are into cycling's equivalent of ultramarathons, century rides, it's also worth considering picking a destination that's about halfway to the mileage goal and just heading there. Once you arrive, you could grab a bite to eat and a coffee, maybe explore some local culture, and then turn around and head for home.

A Virtual Knockout

One area of sports that holds more promise for virtual reality is contact activities that carry the risk of traumatic brain injuries. Andy works closely with several UFC fighters, and their sparring is limited to reduce the number of shots they take to the head. What if a VR simulation came out that offered an immersive experience that mimicked the sensory and motor involvement of real contact, without actual collision forces? Such a game could provide haptic feedback for when a fighter took a punch, but this could be vibrational and nondamaging.

This would enable trainers to lift the limits on sparring, so their charges could get more high-intensity work done in an environment that was engaging and as realistic as possible without the actual contact of gloves hitting their bodies. In addition to transforming the training experience, this would enable fighters to extend their careers and would reduce the chances of their getting degenerative brain conditions later in life. Such technology would have to be used responsibly and sparingly so that fighters still get enough real-world sparring in to recognize the need to defend themselves and have what trainers call "a healthy fear of getting hit."

Think for Yourself

We were born with the instincts to protect ourselves from predators, hunt and kill for food, and find or build shelter. The basic human needs at the bottom of Maslow's hierarchy can all be fulfilled with our innate instincts. So how did we get to a place in which we're relying on gadget-given prompts for when to eat and drink, how hard and long to exercise, and when to sleep? We've delegated decision-making to our gadgets, offshoring our health and humanity in the process.

One quick way to reclaim intuition is to reassert our right to make decisions about our own well-being. You're tired? Sleep. You're hungry? Eat. You're restless? Move. You don't need to wait for your devices to make these choices for you, or to wade through piles of data to confirm what you already know. This might seem elementary, but it's not going to take big, complex solutions to get us back to our real selves. It starts with taking charge of yourself . . . without charging your wearable first.

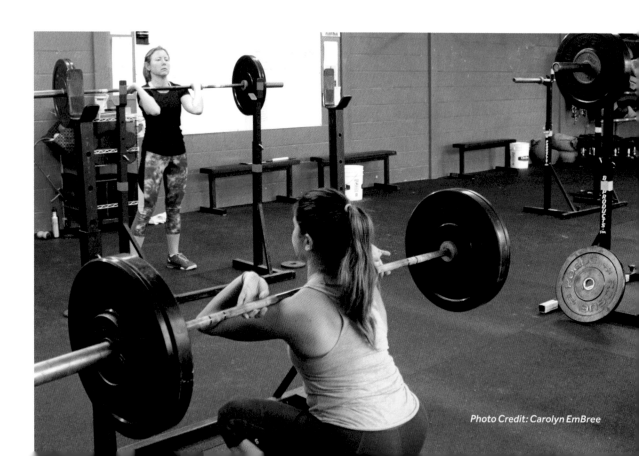

Photo Credit: Carolyn EmBree

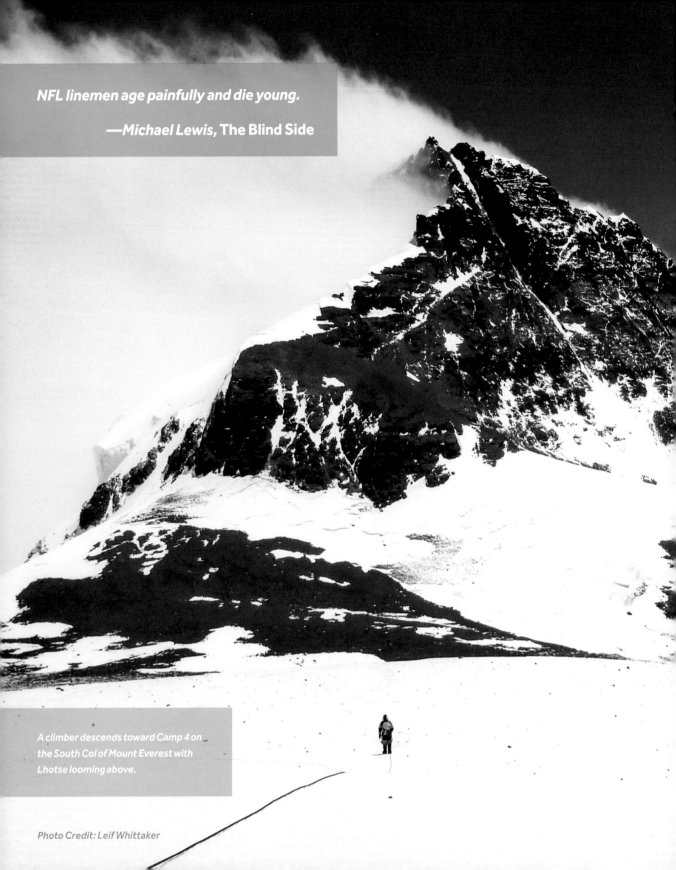

NFL linemen age painfully and die young.

—Michael Lewis, **The Blind Side**

A climber descends toward Camp 4 on the South Col of Mount Everest with Lhotse looming above.

Photo Credit: Leif Whittaker

CHAPTER 6
SEARCHING FOR HEALTH IN FITNESS

Our increasing obsession with team sports has led us to try to emulate the athletic feats of the players we idolize. And to do that, we're going to need big muscles (or so we tell ourselves). Sure, maybe we won't be crushing opponents like J. J. Watt, but we want to be as strong as him, and so we try to squat unholy amounts of weight, as we imagine he does. We might not be able to replicate LeBron James's bowling-ball shoulders, but by golly we're going to do all kinds of presses, flys, and upright rows all the same. Once upon a time, we wanted to emulate the superhero-size action-movie stars of the eighties, like Sylvester Stallone and Arnold Schwarzenegger, so curls became their own religion. Between pro and college sports and movies, we've continued to nurture this desire for both elite performance and aesthetics that are, for most of us mere mortals, unobtainable and unrealistic.

As we've tried in vain to run like Bo Jackson, jump like Michael Jordan, and flex like the Terminator, we've lost sight of health along the way. Most technology that captures real-time information about our bodies is harvesting performance data—distance, altitude gained or lost, split times, and so on. We could apply some information, like heart rate, to our health, but usually we choose to make it all about how we're performing. All we're focused on is how much more we should be doing—which is relayed to us all day by our wearables—and how good that's going to make us look.

When this is the lens through which we view our physical activity, it can cloud the real picture. Certainly, many people who perform well and look good are healthy. Yet many of the athletes whose bodies we admire and whose performances amaze us are profoundly unhealthy. I think of Mark Sisson's revelation in *The Primal Blueprint* that although he had run a 2:18 marathon and looked to be in tip-top shape, he was struggling with chronic inflammation, arthritis in his feet, and multiple other conditions that weren't apparent to anyone who saw his chiseled body or watched him blaze through a race course. He soon realized that the compromises he was making to look and perform like this were no longer worth it and that his super high carb diet, while helping him achieve his short-term goals, was compromising his long-term wellness. The takeaway is that health should always be your primary goal and you shouldn't let looks or technology-driven performance targets become the be-all and end-all. Now let's dive deeper into how a combination of tech, popular culture, and millions of marketing dollars have skewed our perception of what true health is, and how you can find your way back to a more healthful and sustainable mind-set and physical practice.

Weight Loss Isn't Health

One of the primary motivations for people to buy an activity tracker or use a wellness-related app is to lose weight. According to government statistics, two-thirds of American adults are overweight, including the 36.5 percent who are obese. This is clearly a nationwide problem, one that not only ruins individual lives but also costs us $147 billion annually.[104]

It's fairly logical that if you recognize that you're overweight and this is compromising your quality of life, you'd want to find tools that help you take decisive action. So perhaps you buy a wearable or download an app whose maker claims will get you to your target weight. Then you start walking and working toward that ten-thousand-steps-a-day goal. At first, the pounds start coming off. The technology's working!

But then comes the first plateau. You hit a point at which this baseline of recommended activity has stopped leading to weight loss. Should you fail to break through this barrier for a couple of weeks, you'll probably begin to question the effectiveness of the device, and maybe your ability to keep making progress. But the real problem is that you've reduced overall health to a single goal: losing weight. And the only way you've tried to achieve this is through low-level aerobic activity.

Maybe you've also created a new achievement-reward habit: every time you meet your daily steps goal, you treat yourself to a cupcake or a sugary drink at your local coffee shop. Andy's wife has several colleagues who are extremely obese and can't figure out why. She has noticed that although they hit their daily steps goal, they also reward themselves with sugar-laden junk food. In the end, they actually gain weight instead of losing it. This issue is backed up by several recent studies, including one by University of Pittsburgh researchers who found that wearables are less effective for weight loss than old-school diet plans.[105]

This is not to say you should never have any sugar again, but those extra calories can soon add up and chip away at the weight loss. Plus, unless you've combined using your wearable with retooling your overall nutrition, the cupcake might just be a small part of your dietary problem. And if you're like many people, you've also failed to consider how strength training and more strenuous types of activity, not just moving more, might benefit you.

Getting down to a healthy weight and body mass index (BMI) is a noble goal, and if you achieve it, you certainly reduce your risk of heart disease, cancer, and many other diseases. But the $61 billion weight-loss industry has confused the narrative and made us believe that if our weight is what our doctor would recommend, then we're good to go from an overall health perspective.[106] This *can* be true, but very often it isn't. There are plenty of people who are in the "normal" weight range who are profoundly unhealthy.

Some people who meet their weight-loss goal do so using extreme measures that lead to a loss of muscle. Others eat crap, lead chaotic lives that create chronic stress, have broken relationships, and are walking around like zombies on far too little sleep. Just as we can't make the mistake of confusing fitness for wellness, neither should we try to equate weight loss and health. Indeed, one study found that people who are obese yet physically fit (i.e., they have a high VO_2 max) had a

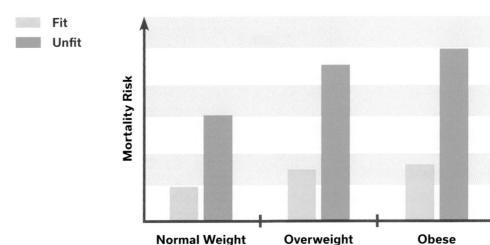

Who Dies First:
"Out of Shape" or "Overweight"

mortality risk 1.6 times the average, but those who are at a normal weight and are unfit (i.e., they have a low VO$_2$ max) have an average mortality risk 3.1 times the average.[107] This isn't to say that being obese is good but rather that fitness is more important than what your bathroom scale tells you, and that being skinny but out of shape can be profoundly unhealthy.

It can also be futile to chase a health goal like lowering blood pressure, which often leads people to obsessively measure their activity, intake of certain foods, and, of course, their blood pressure. A study published in *The Lancet* found that while there's always a lot of media noise about the dangers of high blood pressure and billions of prescriptions are issued annually to manage it, "grip strength was a stronger predictor of all-cause and cardiovascular mortality than systolic blood pressure."[108] This is an example of how strong people generally live longer and healthier lives, and also how monitoring can lead us down the wrong path.

What "Health" Really Means

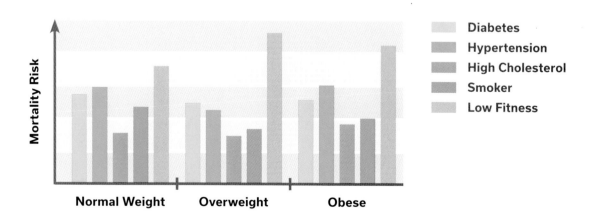

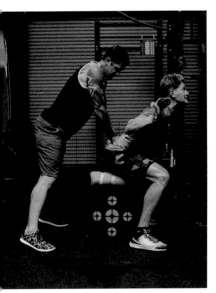

Brian using a combination of technology and his own body to teach an athlete the feel of proper squat positioning.

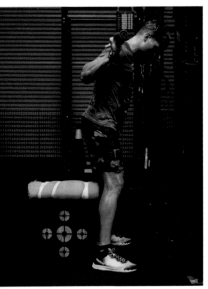

The athlete is then tasked with reproducing the movement without the tactile feedback of Brian's hands. The final progression would be to remove the box.

If you recognize that your blood pressure is too high or your weight isn't where you want it to be, don't fixate on it. Instead, prioritize increasing your activity and sitting less, building muscle, or reaching some kind of performance goal. You will likely reduce your blood pressure, lose fat, and increase lean body mass as a secondary benefit of pursuing such goals, while avoiding the pitfalls of weight loss that many people encounter.

From Beneficial Habit to Harmful Dependence

Merriam-Webster's Dictionary defines a habit as "a settled or regular tendency or practice, especially one that is hard to give up." A habit crosses over into the dangerous territory of addiction when we are psychologically and sometimes physiologically dependent on performing a certain activity and getting the desired outcome. I'll hold up my hand here and admit that I fell into the dependence trap with my breathing practice. I started doing it not for my overall health—which it certainly benefits—but for the feeling of euphoria that it gave me. Think about how you feel if you don't get your first coffee of the day right after you get up. You get twitchy, have no energy, maybe get a headache. It got to the point where my morning was shot if I didn't do my breathing routine first thing. So I had to reexamine my motives, recognize that I had to be able to go through a day without obtaining this oxygen-depletion high, and then reincorporate the breathing into my routine in a less dysfunctional way and with a purer motive.

This is just one example of a possible area of dependence. Coffee is another common one. If it gets to the point that you can't function without it first thing in the morning, try delaying your first cup by a couple of hours until you retrain your body. Then reintroduce it because you like the taste, not because you're addicted to the caffeine. Also examine why you're using your wearable or smartwatch. If it's to keep you honest or help you overcome a motivation issue, then that's okay. But if you're just utilizing it to get validation or because all your friends use similar devices, then perhaps you should reassess your priorities.

The Compromise of Elite Performance

When we watch our favorite pro athletes perform seemingly superhuman feats of athleticism, we assume that they're unbreakable. But just because you do one or a few tasks better than anyone in the world doesn't mean you're healthy. Throwing a ball at a hundred miles per hour a few times every couple of nights is putting your elbow in jeopardy. Putting your head down and charging through a mass of three-hundred-plus-pound bodies for a touchdown is putting your brain in the firing line. Running one hundred miles a week to train for a marathon can destroy your immune system. Just as we shouldn't mistake a "good" body weight for overall well-being, neither should we think that high performers are 100 percent healthy, because they're often not.

"I Can't Breathe, Coach!"

As an emergency-room physician in Florida, Dr. Frank Merritt is on the front line of health care. Through his work with patients, coaching experiences with football players, and personal enjoyment of surfing, Frank has gained uncommonly deep insights into the areas of health, fitness, and performance. Working as part of a multidisciplinary team that included oncologists, behavioral psychologists, nutritionists, and many more specialists as they developed a protocol that would extend the life of his best friend, Jason, who had brain cancer, Frank began to recognize the disconnect between each of these three areas. Determined to narrow the gaps and extend the benefits of what they'd learned during Jason's treatment, the team created a unique seven-dimensional test to assess human vitality, which helps athletes and nonathletes alike find and address their biggest weaknesses in areas such as pulmonary and cardiovascular recovery, adrenal function, and muscle strength and power.

When Frank applied this test to a group of Division 1 football players, he wasn't surprised to see that they were in the ninetieth percentile or above for muscle power and strength. What shocked him was the gulf between this and their cardiopulmonary health, which he found languishing in the fortieth percentile. He then dug deeper and evaluated their heart and lung health separately, something few people even consider doing. Frank discovered that many players' lungs were lagging far behind their hearts, meaning that the big pump in their chest, which was already taxed from carrying all that weight around, was pulling double duty on the cardiovascular front to make up for an inadequate oxygen supply.

Frank believes that part of the problem, aside from the fact that these coaches never train their athletes to improve lung capacity, is the sheer mass that today's football players build in the weight room and at the dinner table. Here's Frank's analogy, which better explains this concept: "Say you put up a fifteen-hundred-square-foot house. You're going to include electrical and HVAC systems that can handle that square

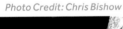

Photo Credit: Chris Bishow

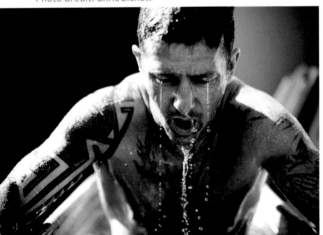

footage. But then you sell that house and the new owner adds on another fifteen hundred square feet. Suddenly you've got a house that's not heated or cooled adequately and has circuits that keep blowing. It's the same with three-hundred-pound players. Their infrastructure hasn't caught up to their size or output. We used to think that high BMI was okay if most of that weight was muscle instead of fat, but we didn't consider the massive internal carbon footprint that such size has on these young men."[109]

To help solve this issue, Frank, Brandon Rager, and their VitalityPro colleagues devised lung workouts that help improve capacity. They also tailored the players' programming so that it simulates playing seventy-two-down games, with each twelve-down possession requiring athletes to maintain 70 percent of their best effort for each play. The results have been amazing, with players who routinely finished last in agility and speed drills becoming top performers and giant linemen who used to tap out of practice after a couple plays being able to stay in and perform at or above that 70 percent mark for the entire drill.

The point here is that so-called fitness testing needs to be far broader than what we've had up until now, and we need to start looking not only at components of health, fitness, and performance but also the biggest discrepancies between all three. With a testing program like the VitalityPro Health Screen, we can use technology appropriately to identify the biggest barriers to success and then create tailored programs for individuals and teams to overcome these. Such an approach is just as applicable to the recreational athlete as it is to the nation's best football players. Tech isn't the solution but a conduit.

Subprime Lending for Your Health

After the financial crash of 2009, as a nation we finally realized that taking out an interest-only loan on a home you can't afford is a bad idea, and that the companies making such loans were building their houses of mammon upon sinking sand. Eventually the bill for that house will come due, and if you've bought a house you can't afford, that bill is disastrous. If we can agree this was foolish, why then do we happily apply subprime thinking to our bodies, giving up future health for short-term performance gains?

Brandon Rager shared with me that when he was playing football for San Diego State University, he used to joke with his teammates about not being able to walk properly or remember anything when they were forty. While they were technically student-athletes, in reality each of these football players considered themselves NFL prospects and were hoping to set their families up for life by making a go of it at the next level.

If you're a legit pro sports prospect, perhaps the risks you're taking—hits to the head, joint deterioration, chronic pain— seem worth it for short-term financial gain, even if the long-term ramifications later call this into question. But if you're a recreational athlete who is taking too much contact, logging too many miles, or putting yourself in a daily hurt locker, what short-term benefits are you getting that outweigh the future issues you're storing up? And is the technology you're using really helping you or just pushing you to go farther, faster, and harder, until you run (or hit, lift, or play) yourself into oblivion?

Consider Michael Lewis's description of a former NFL player in *The Blind Side:* "He limps, but they all limp. One nasty scar runs down his right knee and another lines his left ankle. Former NFL linemen age painfully and die young."[110] If this is how someone might describe you in a few years, how will you answer the simple question, "Was it worth it?" If the answer is likely to be no, then you need to reconsider the goals that you and your gadgets are pushing you toward, and reset them so you don't end up with your health bank foreclosing on a $2 million performance mansion that was far beyond your means.

The Gardener, the Farmer, and the Lineman

Frank realized that while these elite athletes were undoubtedly fit and were able to perform at the highest echelons of competition, they had major limitations in their basic health. This brought him to a question: if these big, strong, fast guys aren't the healthiest population group, then who is? In search of an answer, he began analyzing data on dozens of different sportsmen and women, as well as studies on the overall well-being of various professions and people with all kinds of hobbies. After crunching enough numbers to make him cross-eyed, Frank found that two groups consistently stood out. Triathletes? Nope. Track stars? Guess again. With numerous health and fitness factors taken into account, it was farmers and gardeners who came out on top.

How are these two groups healthier than pro athletes? Frank believes that there are several contributing factors. "Farmers and gardeners are outside most of the time, they're constantly moving, and they have to get into a wide range of positions. Throughout the day they have a few instances of activity that's either high intensity or requires them to lift and carry something heavy. They also have a strong sense of purpose, are part of tight-knit communities, and get satisfaction from the results of a job well done," Frank said.[111] Unsurprisingly, their health has nothing to do with using technology. They don't need to track their activity because they know that it's an ever-present part of their lifestyle. And they are in tune with their own bodies and the soil that they dig in and the crops and plants they grow.

One of the reasons that many of us have lost this elemental connection to ourselves and our environment is because of our tendency to compartmentalize our wellness. "Health and consciousness are indivisible, but we're attempting to separate them into two different things," Laird Hamilton said. "If we just reduce health to all these numbers, where does consciousness come in? We look at a device to tell us we did this or that and how well we did it. But what about our personal monitoring system for each experience, which is how it feels?"[112]

In Pursuit of Balance

There's a line we have to walk between pushing ourselves relentlessly and mercilessly, always in pursuit of more, and allowing ourselves to drift along without challenging ourselves. Both extremes are harmful, and we need to continually check to make sure we're not straying to one side or the other.

Cultivating a Physical Practice

Pavel Tsatsouline, the man who popularized kettlebell training in the US, has said that he hates the term *work out* because it implies that we've literally exhausted all our reserves. He asserts that in his homeland of Russia, people perform their chosen activity in a way that provides just enough stimulus to produce adaptation and no more, so that they're ready to practice their discipline again the next day. But in the West, we go super hard one day and then hobble around until our soreness goes away and we can hammer ourselves again.

I completely agree with Pavel on this. Your physical activity can be challenging. It can be strenuous. But it shouldn't leave you completely "worked out." If you're truly focusing on your overall wellness, you need a physical practice—whether it's kettlebells, like Pavel's, or martial arts, or anything else you find enjoyable—that you can perform every day. Perhaps it's a mix of sports or activities.

Similarly, though there is benefit in high-intensity sessions at a fast pace, you should also be able to find physical and mental value in slower, flowing pursuits, such as holding and carrying weights, practicing tai chi, or even just taking a walk in your local park. We've become too used to applying our go-go-go lifestyle to our physical activity, to our detriment. In the military, there's a saying on this subject: "Slow is smooth. Smooth is fast." I take this to mean that when you rush around, you're going at an unsustainable pace and not paying attention to yourself or what's going on around you. If you're a special operator in combat, this is going to have serious consequences. This mantra also means you should apply enough effort to perform a skill smoothly, but not so much that you sacrifice form for speed or power. This is the exact opposite of the "go faster" messages that our devices give us. To embrace smoothness, we need to set our own pace and find the right rhythm and cadence for our activity.

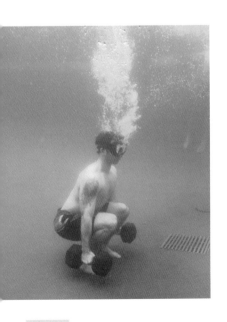

Just Because You Can Do More Doesn't Mean You Should

We may have the capacity to increase load, work rate, or volume, but this doesn't mean it's healthy. One thing no app or device can currently do is measure the total allostatic load—which is a fancy way of saying the amount of stress something places on your body. We can look at individual measurements, whether oxygen saturation and heart rate variability in commercially available technology or muscle breakdown and growth in labs like Andy's at Cal State Fullerton. But even with such tests, we still lack the ability to accurately gauge the overall impact of any session and to make a recommendation for what to do the next day based on this. We're also unable to measure the emotional and cognitive consequences of activity and competition. You might not find a particular activity physically draining, but it might require absolute concentration and so leave you mentally fatigued the next day, or even for a few days.

When we act on our smartwatch's advice to do yet another all-out workout, we often add a stress load to a body and mind that's already overtaxed and underrecovered. In his research, Frank has found that while going too far in a single workout can make our muscles sore for a couple of days, it can take up to two *weeks* for our bodies to fully bounce back from a session that went into overtraining territory. What if your app is pushing you too hard day after day, week after week? Eventually you're going to break down.

The solution is to stop relying on technology to tell you when you're ready to do something or when you need to rest. On those days that you're not sure, you can either turn to a coach who knows how to see patterns in the testing that you are doing, or just do a light-intensity activity, like going on a bike ride with your kids or significant other. You could also do your own heart rate variability or oxygen saturation monitoring for a couple of weeks and sync this up with your perceived energy levels, improvements or dips in performance, and overall well-being. Once you've dialed in the connection between the numbers and your self-awareness, you won't need the technology anymore.

A Point of Diminishing Returns

In the fitness industry, it has become popular to prescribe the minimum effective dose of exercise needed to produce adaptation. This is understandable, as there's no point collecting "junk mileage" that does more harm than good. But often the minimum dose is based on outdated research or blanket averages that work in studies of untrained athletes but not for anyone at a higher level. This is why Andy tests elite athletes to find when they break or, if they don't, to see when a certain stimulus stops producing worthwhile returns. By looking at the extremes that the world's best athletes can go to and identifying when they stop improving, we're better able to work backwards and give more informed recommendations to the rest of us. This is returning exercise physiology to its origins in the Harvard Fatigue Lab.

One way that you can challenge yourself is to push further physically and mentally than you think you can go from time to time, while avoiding overtraining day-to-day and week-to-week. Doing a once-a-year event or taking an adventurous trip that you don't specifically train for once in a while can help you move past technology-imposed parameters and expand your definition of what you're capable of. Maybe that's signing up for a 10k even though you've never run more than a couple of miles, or deciding to do a Tough Mudder or Spartan Race despite the fact you can't climb and don't like the idea of confronting electric wires and icy plunges. Doug Larson, one of Andy's copresenters on the *Barbell Shrugged* podcast, does one thousand burpees every New Year's Day. He doesn't train for it but just jumps right in, literally. Doug makes sure he keeps a sustainable pace and keeps his form perfect, and it takes him about four hours. The experience isn't fun, per se, but he gets a great sense of satisfaction once he's done. If you need extra motivation for your own extreme challenge, sign up with a family member or a group of friends.

The Specialist's Dilemma

From the time they're kids, many athletes become specialists in one sport and become very proficient in it, but they neglect how their body works outside the confines of this single discipline. So basketball players direct all their physical development, cognitive learning, and skill acquisition toward building effectiveness on the hardwood. But unless they play other sports and explore the outdoors as well, they're limiting their proficiency. Focusing exclusively on sports like basketball that involve performing on level surfaces within defined boundaries and against an equal number of similarly skilled opponents means missing out on the varied terrain, freedom, and variety that they would find while snowboarding down a mountain or stand-up paddleboarding in the ocean.

This is not to say that nobody should choose a sport or activity to focus their efforts and time on, but rather that for the sake of their overall well-being, learning, and movement competence, people should also try other active pursuits, some of which should take place outside. This is another area in which fitness technology fails us. Once we've convinced ourselves that we're runners or cyclists, we can get sucked into a netherworld of sport-specific metrics and goals that we might never emerge from. Don't make the mistake of letting your device or app set your agenda or limit you to a single sport. There's so much more out there to enjoy.

Why Are You Here?

Are you following a fitness routine or training for a sport because you want to be or because you feel you have to be? When I first developed the Power Speed Endurance program,

I felt obligated to keep competing in ultramarathons to prove that my methods worked. The problem was that I was also traveling all over the world to host seminars, doing a lot of interviews, and staying up late most nights to make sure everything got done. Add in full commitment to my sport, and you've got a perfect storm for health problems.

It came to the point where I had to just hold up my hands and admit that I couldn't do it all anymore. Simply put, I had to decide between competitive racing and this business that I'd worked so hard to build. I realized that my motivation for continuing the ultras wasn't pure and certainly wasn't beneficial to my mental, physical, or emotional well-being. So I had to let it go.

If you're struggling with health issues or just feeling overwhelmed and run down, ask yourself some questions: Is this training taking more out of me than it's giving back? Why am I doing it? Would my life be better or worse if I did something else? When it comes to a physical practice, you shouldn't do it out of obligation, because you've been doing it since you were a kid, or because it's all you know. If there's no joy in it or it's breaking you down, there's no reason to keep going and you should find something else that makes you happy.

This question of motivation applies to family dynamics, too. Frank Merritt remembers reading about Archie Manning's desire to spend a lot of time with his sons once he retired from the NFL. As a result, he spent hours doing what he did best with them—throwing and catching footballs in the backyard. As a result, Peyton and Eli touched the ball a lot more than they would've if they'd just played Pop Warner football. So indirectly, almost by accident, Archie set them up for their own stellar NFL careers. The lesson here is that if you put a healthy, well-balanced life first, you'll often find fitness and performance along the way.

The Trickle Down

As we've become increasingly fixated on measuring our fitness, it was perhaps inevitable that we'd eventually start pushing the tools that've hooked us onto our children. We've already seen from exposés like Chris Bell and Peter Berg's HBO documentary *Trophy Kids* that our obsession with youth sports achievement has gone way too far. How much worse is it going to get when we're now outfitting our kids— who are already overtaxed with the demands of umpteen after-school activities, traveling for away games, and the weight of our unrealistic expectations—with brightly colored wearables?

It used to be that our parents made sure we got enough movement in our days by sending us outside to play with friends, ride around the neighborhood on our skateboards and bikes, and do whatever the heck we wanted until dinner was ready. But in today's realm of helicopter parenting, when our kids aren't being pushed to a breaking point in youth sports, they're plonked down in front of a video game or one of the six TVs that have colonized most rooms in our houses.

As a result, we're taking them from one high-octane, stress-inducing environment into another. Far too many kids are missing out on the simple joys of creative, unstructured, and minimally supervised play. No wonder so many have attention and personality issues in childhood and serious emotional issues once they've transitioned into our Big Fitness, indoor-only, tech-dominated adult world. We owe it to the next generation to get them outside, unplugged and playing freely, as they should've been all along. Otherwise we're just perpetuating the issues of addiction, obsession, and technology dependence that we're trying to solve for ourselves.

The Lie of Linear Progress

In letting wearables convince us that we must incrementally do more, we've let ourselves be misguided about the nature of real progress. Any elite athlete on the planet can tell you there are days that they backslide in terms of performance, seem to be losing their grasp of a skill they thought they had down, and can't will their bodies to do what their minds know they're capable of. Much as we might want it to be, life is not linear, and neither is our health or fitness. Sometimes we're fighting a cold, trying to repair the damage from an injury, or dealing with a difficult situation at work. These and hundreds of other scenarios, many of which are outside of our control, mean that each day our well-being is a moving target.

This is why we're better off trying to gauge our mood, energy levels, and enthusiasm and adjusting our activity, sleep, and nutrition accordingly, instead of relying on the blanket recommendations of an app, which takes none of these factors into account because they cannot be quantified. So the more we can get in tune with ourselves, the better off we'll be in the long run, even when that means a long run is out of the question.

Finding Your Vitality Age

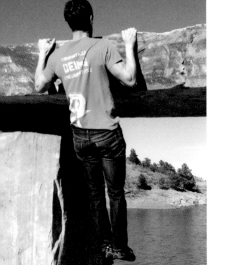

When you go to the doctor for an annual physical, they have a very limited amount of time to try to assess multiple areas of your health, and so they rush through a battery of rudimentary tests that haven't changed in decades. If they find that a level is too high or low, they typically give you very generic and nebulous information about the issue and what to do about it. So if your LDL ("bad") cholesterol is too high, your physician might tell you to "eat healthier." Or if your BMI is above average, you might be advised to "exercise more."

The shortcomings in such testing and the intangible, nonspecific recommendations that follow prompted Frank Merritt and his partners at VitalityPro to look for a better path to true health. After wading through mountains of research and consulting with specialists as diverse as physical therapists, behavioral psychologists, and nutritionists, they came up with a seven-part health screen founded on evidence-based best practices. The VitalityPro screen assesses cardiovascular and pulmonary health, mobility, body composition, and muscular fitness and assigns a relative age for each. Twenty is ideal and eighty is the worst score. The assessment then aggregates the category scores to generate an overall vitality age. Individuals are then given protocols to improve on the areas in which they're lacking.

Certain aging factors can't be controlled (such as those related to genetics), but the VitalityPro team believes that many are correctable and can be improved through targeted health interventions that don't involve pharmaceuticals, surgery, or any of the other drastic measures that are often prescribed when a doctor finds a patient to be in pain or deficient in some area. By identifying detrimental factors that are aging people beyond their chronological age, Frank, Brandon, and their team are able to improve quality of life and remove roadblocks to overall well-being. Once someone's health is better, then they can build fitness and performance on a sounder foundation.

The VitalityPro team uses technology in the diagnostic stage and, where necessary, as educational tools that help people better understand the link between what's happening in their body and how they feel. But there is no app or device that offers a magic bullet. What's needed is a commitment to overall health and daily awareness of what's working, what's not, and how we can do better.

We were not chasing medals; medals were just the tangible rewards. We were chasing excellence, and we achieved it often, and, in the process, gained even more: an appreciation for each other that would sustain itself long after his swimming career ended.

—Coach Bob Bowman on working with Michael Phelps for twenty-one years[113]

Photo Credit: Jennifer Cawley

CHAPTER 7
COACHING 2.0: TECH AS A TOOL, NOT A TASKMASTER

Usain Bolt. Katie Ledecky. Mikaela Shiffrin. All of these stars are at the pinnacle of their sports, yet none of them can do without the daily guidance of their expert coaches, not to mention the physical therapists, masseurs, nutritionists, and other support staff who help them reach even greater heights every time an Olympic final, world championship, or World Cup rolls around. So at what point did the rest of us decide that cutting coaches out of the picture and replacing them with a wearable was a good idea? You're trading years of expertise for a device that advises you based on an unsensing, unknowing algorithm. Do you think the best athletes in the world would entrust their success to the whims of a machine? No. Then why would you?

Coaching or technology doesn't have to be an either/or choice. But while coaching without technology can provide lasting value, technology without coaching does not, at least not if your goal is to improve health, fitness, and performance over the long term. A discerning coach will use devices discerningly when they're necessary. But they're employed as part of a broader solution, not as a cure-all.

In this chapter, we'll explore the pitfalls of trying to replace a real coach with an electronic substitute, whether that's a fitness tracker, online app, or "coach in your ear" that uses an algorithm to try to connect a small number of biometrics with how much longer and harder you should train. We'll also look at the intangibles coaches offer that no technology can replicate, from an expert eye to mentoring to a holistic approach to improving your lifestyle, and more. You'll see how it doesn't need to be an either/or choice when it comes to coaching and fitness tech; you can take a hybrid approach in which the coach is the guide, arbiter, and teacher who uses heart rate monitoring, biomarkers, and other tech-derived insights as tools to help improve your self-knowledge, awareness, and technique.

Let Your Coach Be Your Guide

In the age of the quantified self, we've taken to outsourcing fitness and health guidance to devices and software. Whether intentional or not, this has led to the devaluation of coaching. As technology temporarily relieves us from our decision fatigue and the two-way investment that coaching entails, many people have decided that a wearable is a viable option, or even a better one. Nothing could be further from the truth.

In fact, the eyes of an expert coach who has amassed years of experience can spot flaws in our technique far more readily and instinctually than any piece of clothing with a chip embedded in it or four-dimensional video analysis, and can find problems in our programming that no algorithm would ever detect. This is why I believe that once the backlash against outsourcing our wellness to technology has had time to gather momentum, we'll see a resurgence in engagement with coaches and trainers.

Another factor will be the realization that we need greater connection with other people and less with the gadgets that have isolated us. But this can only happen if we recognize that our wearables and smart devices will always have limitations and leave gaps that only human beings, with their combination of experience, instincts, and judgment, can truly fill. In connecting with people instead, we'll tap into a deeper well of performance than any technology can offer.

That said, coaches can make effective use of the latest technology within their evidence-based programming approach. When my wife, Erin, decided to come out of competitive retirement to help a friend whose rowing pairs partner dropped out due to injury, she was many miles away from her coach. So she used the Concept2 rowing machine to monitor her workouts, took a photo of her stats after each session, and sent it to her coach to show how she'd done against that day's targets. This proved very effective at overcoming the physical distance between Erin and Tom and enabling him to assess her progress and make on-the-fly adjustments to her personalized program as needed.

So my point is that we shouldn't cut the cord on technology completely but rather reintegrate it into sensible, holistic coach-athlete relationships as just another arrow in our quiver, instead of the main thing that monitors, directs, and instructs us.

Believe What You See

When Andy started working with some UFC fighters a few years back, he watched them practice, and when they asked him what their main weakness was he told them simply, "You're not producing enough power and you're not explosive." Perhaps predictably, these tough young men, all hopped up on testosterone after a couple of hours of grappling, were incredulous. "Not powerful enough?" one of them scoffed. "I've had seven knockouts in my last ten fights!"

It wasn't until Andy invited the fighters up to his Cal State lab for testing that he was able to convince them that he was correct. He had them jump on a force plate that recorded their power production and reaction time and displayed these as colored curves on a big monitor. Andy then overlaid the same metrics from NFL players and showed how they produced far more power and did it much faster than the mixed martial artists. "Once they saw it with their own eyes, they believed everything I told them after that," Andy said. This shows how technology can be used by a coach to gain buy-in from his or her athletes, and to present an abstract concept (like "power" or "explosiveness") in a simple, graphical way.

The Value of Tech-Enabled Cues

When you're a novice, it can be hard to understand certain coaching cues because if you haven't done something (or done it properly) before, you don't know how the desired action or technique is supposed to feel. Without this anchor point, the coach is speaking a language that you can't decipher. This is where mobile apps and old-school objects alike can come into play. Say your coach notices that you round your back when you squat, which is limiting your performance and putting you at risk of injury. She tells you that you're doing it but you don't notice that you are, and you're not even sure what "rounding" means in this sense. You certainly don't know what it feels like at the point that your spine starts to curve abnormally.

In this situation, your coach could get you to squat next to a mirror and have you watch yourself so that you see the point at which your back starts to round. Now you understand what that term means and how it looks when you lose control of your posture. Or maybe the mirror isn't cutting it because you're too distracted and can't multitask between looking in the mirror and trying to focus on your technique. In this case, the coach could use an inexpensive yet effective app like

Coach's Eye to record your next squat while you concentrate on performing the movement. When you're done, she comes over to you, plays the video in slow motion, and shows you how and when your spine started curving. Such apps sometimes have colored lines that show the ideal path for a limb or motion segment and can show where you're going wrong.

Once you've seen the point at which your spine begins to round, the coach now shouts "Stop!" once you reach it during a squat. She then asks you to focus on how your back and hips are feeling when the curve kicks in. Once you can home in on how the rounding feels when it happens and you understand the consequences—a sore back the next day at best, a blown disc at worst—you've developed the body awareness to identify the problem yourself.

The next step is selecting and implementing an appropriate solution. Your coach decides that your back starts rounding because you lose tension in your abs as you're on the way down into the bottom portion of your squat. So she gives you the simple cue, "Make your abs as hard as a rock." You then perform the squat with that thought in mind and squeeze your midsection muscles as hard as you can throughout the movement. Now the coach uses the mirror or app again to show you the difference, and boom! No more rounding. She has you do a few more squats to make sure the new, better pattern becomes ingrained, and the session is done for the day. Later, she e-mails you the before-and-after video with the subject line, "Make those abs as hard as a rock." This reminds you what to do next time and helps you commit the lesson from your short-term memory to long-term.

If you're a more advanced athlete who is familiar with the skills you're working on, your coach might be able to skip ahead to telling you what to do, or add in some imagery, such as telling a basketball player to "make your follow-through like a goose neck." But if you're a novice, your coach would be better off using a visual aid first so you can see the problem, then have you feel it with a kinesthetic (or movement- and

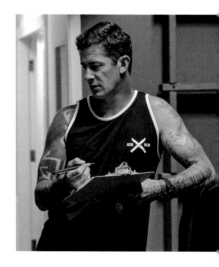

feeling-based) cue and finally give the appropriate auditory pointer to self-correct it.

In such a progression, technology is not a crutch but an instructional prop that provides instant feedback and enables you to feel and then act in response to your heightened awareness. In the last stage of the process, the smartphone and app are set aside because you can now identify and fix the error without them. This means that you can self-correct not only in the weight room without your coach there but also whenever you need to squat in your sport. This level of finely tuned physical awareness should be what you're striving for with every movement.

The New Laws of Remote Coaching

When he first started consulting with individual athletes, Lenny Wiersma insisted on meeting them in person. But as time went on and his reputation grew, he started attracting clients from all over the world, and even with the best frequent flyer miles account of all time, he could no longer restrict himself to only face-to-face meetings. Enter Facetime and Skype.

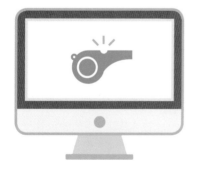

I was initially very skeptical of video conferencing with clients. But I started to find that it could give me insight into my athletes that I wouldn't have had otherwise. While some people dial in remotely, most talk to me from their homes. One time I was on a video call with a college athlete and noticed a Captain America poster on his dorm room wall behind him. I thought that was a little odd as college athletes don't usually have superhero posters up, and he was a foreign student, so it wasn't a patriotism thing. I asked him about it and found that he used the metaphor of the shield to remind him that he could deflect criticism and pressure from others. This spawned a whole in-depth discussion that we never could've had if the technology hadn't given me an inside view of his world.[114]

The usefulness of video isn't limited to live interaction. Tim Ferriss has found it beneficial to upload videos of his workouts to Dropbox, so his gymnastics coach, Chris Sommer, can monitor his progress and fix mechanical errors. "I think that my coach's video reviews have certainly helped me to develop a better awareness of my movement and how what I think I'm doing often deviates dramatically from what I'm actually doing."[115]

Technology can also allow coaches to create a network for other practitioners who are applying their system and methods. A master coach or founder of a system could benefit from the same video streaming that I've used to monitor my athletes, periodically evaluating the quality of the experiences others are creating for their clients. This can help entrepreneurs scale their businesses without the time and financial costs of traveling all over the globe to meet with employees and coaches face-to-face.

Expertise and Experience

One of the most important things coaches offer is the benefit of their long experience and earned expertise. Whatever concern you have or topic you're interested in, chances are, they've either encountered it before or have the education and knowledge to guide you through it in a way that no wearable or app ever could.

Curators Wanted

One of the huge advantages that the internet provides is the availability of information on health and performance. Thirty years ago, you'd have had to enroll in a college program or go to a library and binge-read impenetrable, jargon-filled textbooks (which were often woefully out-of-date) to learn more. Now all you need is a Wi-Fi-enabled device and a web browser. Yet this ease of access is in some ways a double-edged sword. Yes, we now have millions of pages of information just milliseconds away. But who has the time to sift through it all and determine what's valid and what's useless? If you go to any of the main research websites (such as Research Gate, PubMed, or Academia.edu) and enter any search term, thousands of studies will pop up. Where do you even start?

What we need isn't more info or data but greater discernment. Just as news aggregation sites supply a digestible overview of the latest happenings in politics and world affairs, we need more curators to sift through the latest evidence-based practices and practice-based evidence and present the best of it to us, and then to help us apply it to our individual physiology. This is another void that coaching can fill.

Another useful resource is podcasts. Andy's *Body of Knowledge* and *Barbell Shrugged* podcasts, *Radiolab*, *The Tim Ferriss Show*, *The Joe Rogan Experience,* and *Ben Greenfield Fitness* are just a few of many that feature some of the world's leading scientists and top performance experts. The best place to start is to seek out a podcast host whom you consider a thought leader, or to check out the websites and social-media feeds to see which shows some of the experts have appeared on as guests. Still can't find what you're looking for? Ask your coach and training partners for guidance.

Peaking vs. Adaptation

Another limitation of fitness tracking is that the technology doesn't understand your goals. If you're training to peak for a single event, the stimuli and recovery your body needs are different from those required to just get you to adapt— whether that means building muscle, improving endurance, or whatever your aim is. If you're targeting adaptation, you need to overload your body so that it recognizes the stimulus and responds to it by prompting muscle growth, improved cellular efficiency, and so on.

During such an adaptation cycle, your resting heart rate or heart rate variability numbers might be screaming at you to stop and rest. But to get the overload you need, you actually *should* train. The opposite might be true if you're trying to peak for a race, fight, or competition. In this case, relying on the one-size-fits-all algorithm of a machine could very well give you the wrong advice, compromising your goals.

This is another area where coaching comes into play. Decades of experience and gut-level understanding of your motivation and physiology will enable a seasoned coach to tell you when to push and when to back off. Metrics can help, but the big picture encompasses far more than the numbers alone.

The Master and the Apprentice

Back in the day, there was no such thing as a hack or a crash course. If you wanted to learn how to do something well, you studied for years under a master in the craft, whether that was thatching roofs, laying bricks, or forging iron. The same is still true in martial arts but, sadly, in few other walks of life. While many of the trades that apprentices learned a couple of hundred years ago have vanished or are heading that way, the coach-athlete relationship offers one way to recapture the lasting benefits of learning from a master. From Mr. Miyagi and Daniel in *Karate Kid* to Yoda and Luke Skywalker in the *Star Wars* saga to Frankie Dunn and Maggie Fitzgerald in *Million Dollar Baby*, we're drawn to tales of someone older imparting wisdom to his or her young protégé. Perhaps this is appealing because so few of us have experienced the benefits of such a partnership.

With technology, it's now easier than ever before for masters to keep their apprentices accountable. A fitness tracker is impartial and doesn't care who you are—it records that either you did the same workout as your teammates or you didn't. Andy's mixed martial arts coach has his athletes text him photos of their resting heart rates each morning, knowing that a huge spike means that either the previous day's load was too great or the fighter hasn't recovered sufficiently to go right into another similarly demanding session. He has developed this intuition by working with dozens of fighters over many decades. In such a scenario, technology can play a role in the master-apprentice relationship, as long as it's used with restraint and purpose.

The True Meaning of Mentorship

Fitness technology can measure many of our physical qualities. But what it can't do is quantify our ever-changing mind-set and emotional state. When he started working with high school football players, Brandon Rager used to think an athlete was dogging it or being soft if he performed poorly on the practice field or had an off day in the weight room. But as he matured as a coach and got to know his players more as people, he started seeing that such dips in performance were frequently tied to some kind of off-field issue. A good coach makes the effort to build in-depth relationships with their athletes and builds up trust so they feel they can share problems and ask for advice when they need it. Enabling athletes to fulfill their athletic potential is certainly important, but helping them to live fuller lives is even more rewarding. There's no app for that!

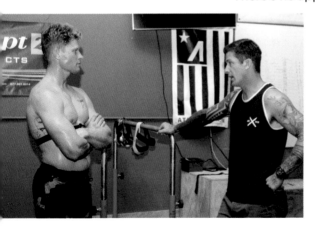

Now let's examine how the role of the coach can go far beyond simply improving physical performance. A truly effective coach doesn't just know his or her sport inside out and know how to create training programs that lead to excellence in it but is also an expert communicator, a psychologist, and an educator. The best coaches don't eschew technology completely but use it discriminately to empower athletes and make them more self-reliant and independent.

Thirty Rowers, Eight Seats, One Coach

Long before Erin Cafaro became my wife, she was one of my athletes. This gave me the privilege of looking inside her preparations for two Olympics, which was a valuable part of my education. The four-year cycle that Olympians operate within is incredibly grueling. Yes, they do create lasting, lifelong friendships with some teammates. But the competition is fierce and unrelenting. There are thirty rowers competing for eight seats in one boat, so there's bound to be some sniping as each person tries to stake their claim to one of those precious seats. To be honest, I've never witnessed more drama in my entire life, let alone my coaching career.

You'd think that the head coach would get pulled into the rivalries, the seesaw relationships, and the tears. But not in the case of this women's eight. Throughout both Olympic cycles, I was amazed by how Coach Tom Terhaar managed to stay above all of that and remain focused on the task at hand: getting his athletes ready and prepared and picking those who would comprise yet another world-beating boat. He'd come in every day with the same all-business attitude, even when the emotional tension reached fever pitch in the boathouse. His no-nonsense, pragmatic attitude was what held the squad together and enabled him to push the ladies to their limits but not beyond them. It was the most impressive display of team coaching imaginable. Tom reinforced how crucial the attitude and demeanor of a coach is, and the importance of letting athletes figure things out on their own.

Tom also had, and probably still has to this day, a skeptical attitude toward technology. Yes, the team did some testing to establish lactate and aerobic thresholds, which allowed him to create tailored training programs. And he encouraged Erin and the others to snap pictures of their Concept2 rowing machine monitors on days that required them to be indoors instead of out on the water. But what he realized was that tech is just one of many interconnected means to an end—it wasn't the focal point of training. This was just another lesson in his coaching master class.

Tom made sure technology was a valuable tool because it was part of a holistic approach to training that wasn't just about the numbers. "First I learned how to use the Concept2 monitor to get instant feedback and to see how certain changes I'd make affected my speed," Erin said. "When Tom introduced heart rate monitoring, it was a useful way for him to guide sixty athletes who he didn't get to spend enough time with, and helped me better understand how my pulse corresponded to my perceived effort level. Using fitness technology can become a game to see who can get the highest numbers, but our goal was to become more efficient—to generate the most speed and power while keeping our heart rates low."

That said, Tom never used technology for its own sake during Erin's preparation for the Olympics and was quick to abandon methods that didn't prove beneficial. "At one point we started using 'smart' oars that showed the power curve for each rower's stroke," Erin said. "If there was a dip in the curve it was meant to show a disconnection from the oars and identify areas of inefficiency. But when Tom started looking at the numbers, he found that some of the lower-level athletes had the best-looking force charts. The best rower on the team had the worst. That's when he decided to stop using this measurement, because the numbers didn't correspond to what was actually happening in the boat."[116]

Empowering Self-Care

In some sections of the coaching community, there has always been a degree of protectionism: coaches are reluctant to openly share their knowledge with their clients or the wider world for fear that they'll lose business and revenue. But the best coaches I know—including Kelly Starrett, Mike Burgener, and Tom Terhaar, to name just three—willingly answer questions, fully disclose what they've learned in interviews, and create videos, books, and other media that give the public the same kind of access as the people these experts work with daily.

To me, it's the job of every coach to empower their athletes with the know-how to learn and grow on their own. In my case, this means playing the role of teacher so that you have at least a rudimentary understanding of your own physiology and how this impacts your training, mobility, preparation, recovery, nutrition, hydration, and every other aspect of your overall wellness. If coaches want the best for their athletes, they have to encourage their independence, like a parent teaching a child how to drive. Just as Mom and Dad know that their kid is eventually going to be on the road by themselves (breathe, parents of new drivers), so too must coaches recognize that they can't be present for every moment of the day. This means that you, the athlete, are going to have to learn how to do things on your own.

With regards to technology, coaches must demonstrate appropriate use, encouraging their athletes to use wearables only when necessary and helping them pay better attention to their instincts at all other times. The coach should act like an Outward Bound guide whose aim is to educate a group of teenagers so that they better understand their environment and how they can interact with it safely, responsibly, and independently.

Lifestyle Programming

One of the issues with fitness apps, trackers, smartwatches, and the rest is that they attempt to carve up our lives like pieces of your grandma's pumpkin pie at Thanksgiving— activity is here, nutrition's over there, and so on. The same is true in medicine. If your doctor thinks you have a heart issue, they'll refer you to a cardiologist. If your foot hurts, off you go to a podiatrist. This segmentation and the way that our devices collect and present information give the false impression that each area is distinct and contained in its own neat little box: "exercise," "fitness," "recovery," and so on. Not so. The phrase "Everything is everything" might be overused, but when it comes to our health it's also valid. If you recover insufficiently, you're not going to process food or absorb fluids optimally. Push yourself every day in the gym? You're going to get sick more often because your nervous system, which is intertwined with immune response, is overtaxed.

This is where an experienced coach can come alongside you. They're not just going to look at the exercise you're doing, the food you're eating, or the sleep you're getting (or not, in many cases); they will piece all of this together to create a big-picture view. Instead of trying to improve your overall well-being with marginal gains through this app or that pair of shoes, they'll try to identify lifestyle mistakes that are holding you back and that, once remedied, will yield huge benefits. No matter what Silicon Valley tells you, there's no device or software program that can do this as well as a coach.

Taking the Long View

One of the benefits of fitness-focused technology is that it gives us instant feedback on our cadence, distance, and more. But that immediacy is also one of its limitations, as those numbers are constantly morphing and anytime you look at your wearable you are only getting a snapshot relevant to that exact moment in time.

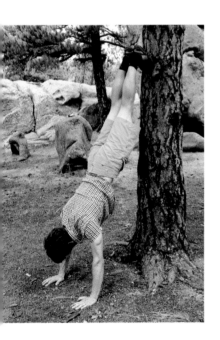

This is why a coach can be helpful in playing the long game. They might want to know how you perform in each session, but only within the context of broader goals and your overall health. They know that it's not good to have a session that looks excellent on paper (or, indeed, on a screen) but really sets you back because you used poor technique or put yourself in harm's way. An expert coach knows how to look at the quality of each session and notice indicators that don't show up on a tracker or that make its numbers useless. Perhaps you PR'd your dead lift but your knees caved in while you were doing it. In this case, your wearable would congratulate you on a job well done, while your coach would know that you gave up proper form and risked injury. He or she can explain to you that this isn't sustainable and what the consequences are when you compromise tomorrow for the sake of today. Such insight requires a human perspective.

You're More Than an Algorithm

App developers are falling over themselves to produce software that creates diet plans, training programs, and recovery protocols based on the latest and, supposedly, greatest algorithms. Yet no matter how many people's data they're using to create lines of best fit, they can't escape the fact that physiology is and always will be highly individualized. Say you have two female skiers who are both twenty-five, weigh 150 pounds, and are five feet eight inches tall. An app would likely conclude that they're the same and spit out identical programs for them. And yet if you dig deeper, you'll find that these women have different injury histories, body compositions, and many other differences that aren't evident in rudimentary and reductionist data and would impact how they respond to the app's programming. So if they both stick to the plan, one might progress in leaps and bounds while the other stagnates.

This is another area that a good coach can help in, as they can dig deeper into an athlete's physiology, history, culture, and background and then combine this knowledge with their prior experience to create effective, sustainable, and tailored programs that don't rely on algorithmic assumptions and one-size-fits-all recommendations. Getting to know an athlete means going beyond what the numbers tell us.

The Progress Report Risk

Users of some wearables get a weekly "progress report" so they can see how they're doing with step totals, total exercise time, heart rate, and so on. Some gear makers also enable users to select several people to compare themselves with.

The issue with this, and why I used quotes around the term *progress report*, is that technology can reduce progress to increasing daily and weekly totals.

For people who've been sedentary for years, such reports can provide a little short-term motivation, and some people can find welcome accountability and encouragement in comparing themselves with a group of friends who are at a similar level. But for those who are already active, the usefulness of weekly graphs and charts soon diminishes. Anyone who is above a novice level in a sport needs to shift their focus from how *much* they're doing to how *well* they're doing it. Otherwise they get caught in the high-mileage, high-volume arms race that has burned out, injured, and forced the retirement of all too many athletes. Often, it takes the expertise of a coach to analyze the kind of numbers that wearables deliver to your inbox daily, weekly, or monthly, put these into context, and see how the quantity of the work you're doing is positively or negatively impacting its quality. The data can provide some useful baselines, but it typically takes the experience and broad view of a coach to draw meaningful conclusions from it and to make these actionable.

Ryan Hall, one of the best American marathoners of his generation, is a prime example. He stepped away from elite-level running in 2015 because all those steps had left him broken, at the ripe old age of thirty-three. Too many miles had led not just to injury and a lack of a new personal best since 2008 but also to chronic fatigue and low testosterone—telltale signs that an athlete's nervous system can no longer cope with their training volume.[117] This is not a knock on Hall, who just became a victim of a numbers-obsessed, more-is-better system. The issues that forced him to quit aren't just occurring at the world-class level but are also increasingly prevalent among recreational athletes.

Since he stopped logging high mileage, Hall has put on forty pounds of lean muscle while embracing the strength training that he worried would make him too bulky during his competitive career. Asked about his new routine by *Runner's*

World, he said, "I feel like it's giving life to my body instead of taking it away. Now I can go run and not feel fatigued and feel good. But I'm also doing so much less running-wise than I ever have—like, 12 miles a week compared to 12 miles a day."[118]

The Surprising Importance of David Puddy

If your car is running hot or making a weird noise, you won't take it just anywhere but to a mechanic whom you know and trust to give you a fair price—like David Puddy in *Seinfeld*. Even though modern mechanics use sophisticated diagnostic systems to evaluate your computer-controlled vehicle, the machines alone aren't enough, or else we'd have repair shops with no actual humans in them. Instead, the mechanic must know which tests to run on what parts of your car, and then how to interpret the results. Once they know the problem, they have to look up the required part and order it, and then they need to have the know-how to install it just so. Indeed, Frank Merritt insists on going to a mechanic who rides in the car with him when his car has an issue, so he can point out the weird rattling noise that a computer program would fail to pick up.

This is similar to how an effective coach uses technology to evaluate your capabilities and problems and find solutions to them. And just as you can't put a Ford Fiesta carburetor in a Ferrari—the parts, tires, and tune-ups need to be specific to the brand and vehicle—the same goes in coaching. Technology might well be used to run a diagnostic check, but it's years of expertise, the coach's knowledge of your body and lifestyle, and his or her ability to interpret your data that's going to make all the difference. Though you might initially worry that you can't afford a coach, it's the best way to achieve lasting improvements. In the long run, it will actually save you money by reducing or eliminating injury-related bills from physical therapists, chiropractors, and orthopedists, not to mention allowing you to avoid endless experimentation with every new gadget that hits the market.

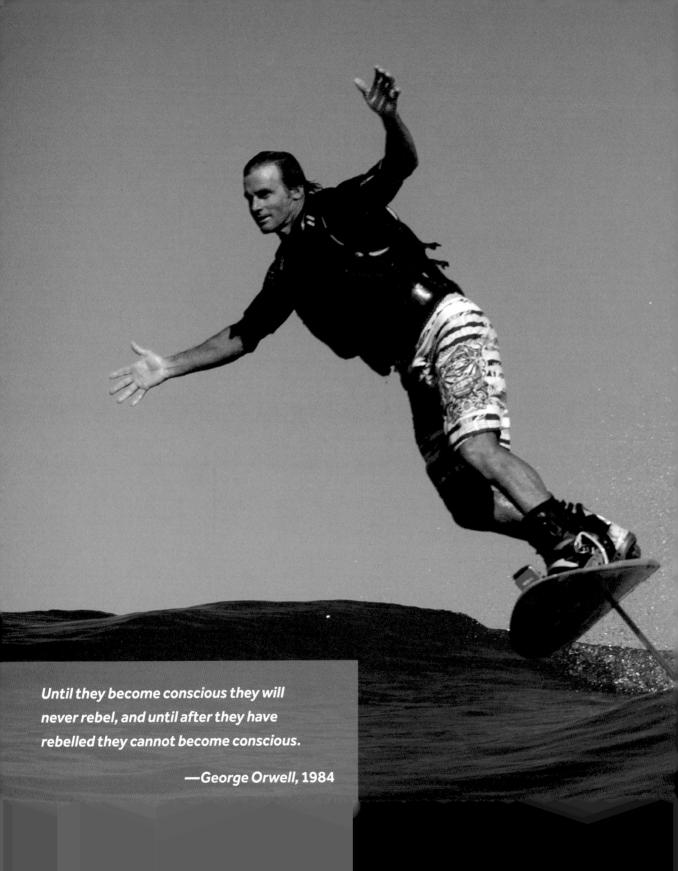

Until they become conscious they will never rebel, and until after they have rebelled they cannot become conscious.

—George Orwell, 1984

CHAPTER 8
BETA TESTING THE SELF-DRIVING ATHLETE

Now that we've looked at many of the limitations of technology, why it shouldn't replace your coach, and how your usage habits drive your behavior, it's time to move further into how best to progress beyond device dependence. In this chapter, we'll examine what it looks like to become more aware, more intentional, and more connected to the world around you, and what kind of disconnection from your gadgets this is going to require.

Becoming Aware: Natural Intelligence

One of the most profound quotes I've come across in the past couple of years comes from the Indian mystic Lalla. She wrote, "The only offering you can make to God is your increasing awareness." Now, not to get too spiritual on you, but I think that no matter what your religious background—or even if you don't have one—you can agree that by increasing your level of consciousness, you can participate more fully and richly in the world around you.

As we've covered elsewhere in this book, technology can be a valid aid that helps us become more aware of our bodies and minds. But once we've used it for this purpose and we can tie feelings, mood, emotion, and energy levels to certain states and events that occur within our activity of choice, it's time to let our gizmos collect dust on the shelf until we need them again to fine-tune our instincts. If you're continually plugged into a device, it's impossible to use anywhere close to your full natural intelligence. Once you get to the point that you must have your wearable with you (and if you don't, you feel "naked" and vulnerable, as did 45 percent of survey respondents when they took off their wearable), you're paying more attention to it than to yourself, other people, or your environment.[119] By trying to reduce our active experiences to numbers, we've diminished our awareness to the point that we've become numb. If this sounds like you, you're overdue for a wearables fast and need to quit cold turkey until you relearn how to feel.

Hunger and Thirst? There's an App for That

Two of the most elemental instincts we have are hunger and thirst. Knowing when we need to eat and drink has helped keep us going as a species. But now some techies have apparently decided that such hardwired survival instincts are

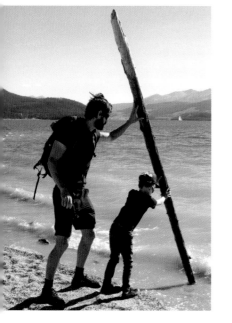

inadequate. So they've come up with gadgets that will *tell* us when we need to eat or drink.

Now, the debate on whether you should "drink to thirst" is ongoing, and we know from recent research on ketones (molecules produced during fat metabolization that the body uses for fuel) by Dominic D'Agostino and others that our bodies can run on very little fuel for days. Most physiology textbooks agree that if we have enough fat in our body, we can, theoretically, exercise for thirty days straight without eating. In one extreme case, someone successfully completed a 382-day fast (albeit with limited food intake, not complete food deprivation).[120] But regardless of how long you could go without eating, completely contracting out our physiology's decision-making is going too far beyond what current technology is capable of.

Instead, we need to be more mindful of our hydration and nutrition and how these affect our performance and health. Fasting periodically is one way to dial in this area of your life. Another is to try different amounts and types of food and beverages at various times of day and before, during, and after activity and see what effect these have on your energy levels, output, and recovery. Also, pay attention to how your productivity and emotions are affected by dietary changes and fluid levels. Then go with what you know works best, not what an app tells you to eat or drink.

You could start with an eighteen-hour fast. Eat a normal meal four to five hours before you go to bed, then don't eat again for another thirteen or fourteen hours—if you get eight hours of sleep, that can mean just skipping breakfast and eating a regular lunch five or six hours after you wake up. If you do it fairly easily the first time, try stretching your willpower by going to twenty-four, then thirty-six, and eventually forty-eight hours without food, making sure you drink water to stay hydrated. You'll start to learn the difference between eating to satisfy hunger and eating merely out of habit or because you're bored. If you're feeling daring, work out as usual during that time. As long as you don't psych yourself out, my guess is that you won't perform much worse than normal, if at all. And here's a pro tip for that initial eighteen-hour fast: try it on a day that you're super busy. That way you won't be as fixated on the lack of food as you would be on a slow day at work or when you're at home all day.

You Can't Weigh Self-Control

As people turn to technology in an attempt to control their calorie intake, limit their portion sizes, and ensure they're eating a balanced diet, we're seeing not just apps that tell us if a meal is healthy or unhealthy but also "smart" forks and storage containers that try to limit food consumption. However, despite the novelty of such devices, their makers are really misunderstanding how willpower and habits work.

Initially, someone who has just shelled out a bunch of money for a new appetite control tool will be eager to get some kind of return on their investment. If they've told other people about the purchase, they'll also want to give a glowing review to justify their decision. But after the fork has beeped at them a few times to tell them that they should stop eating or the storage container's display has reminded them that there are still two days to go until they can have another piece of that oh-so-good chocolate cake, the novelty will likely wear off— particularly if the user is still hungry once the technology has said no. Then there's the possibility of substituting the chip-controlled fork with a regular one, or simply prying the lid off the container to get that cake.

If we get rid of one habit, we need to replace it with another that yields a similar feeling. The rush of neurochemicals you experience when you indulge in that creamy pasta (with a regular fork, of course) or when the sugar in that irresistible cake hits your bloodstream can't be merely cut off. We have to put some other kind of reward in its place.

The rush of dopamine and other feel-good chemicals produced when we move mirrors the rush produced when we consume food we like—but without the blood glucose crash that all that cake frosting leads to. So if you're trying to limit your portion size and are tempted to overindulge, you could move instead of eat. This is why some teachers who are trying to get sugar out of their classrooms offer students an extra movement break instead of candy when they ace a test or help clean up. Andy's wife, Natasha, has a classroom policy that kids aren't allowed to bring any junk food to school. If they do, she sends it back home with a note and a list of healthy exchange items. Instead of creating a reward system based around sugary treats, she gives the kids more free time to play. Now that they're used to it, the three- and four-year-olds in her class go crazy when a parent tries to sneak cookies into their child's backpack and start yelling, "No cookies at school!"

Also, you'd be amazed how quickly your usual sugar cravings go away after going sugar-free for a couple of days (no added sugar, though the naturally occurring sugar in fruit and vegetables are fine) or after an eighteen-hour fast. Take away something that you'll really miss in your daily routine, something whose absence hurts for the first couple of days. After a few days, you'll notice that you have much more self-control.

Connecting Food, Tech, and Feeling

One way that technology can be used to help modify eating habits in a more helpful way than using smart forks or vault-like containers is by connecting feelings and mood with physiology. Say that one day you think that those Pop-Tarts you've been stuffing in the toaster before you dash out the door each morning are probably not the healthiest choice. You decide to run a quick and easy self-experiment to find out if this instinct is correct. On Monday, you use a cheap blood glucose monitor, which you can buy at any drugstore or supermarket, right when you get up. Then you eat your Pop-Tarts (strawberry, naturally), wait a few minutes, and check your glucose level again. It has spiked way up. You record the

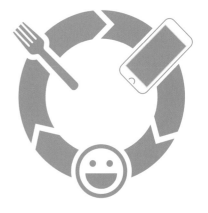

before and after levels in a food log app and add how you felt before and after breakfast. You do the same an hour later, once you've arrived at work. At that point your glucose level has dropped significantly, with your energy levels plummeting right along with it.

The following morning, you try eating a cheese and vegetable omelet instead and repeat the process of writing down your blood glucose levels and how you feel before and after breakfast and an hour later. You find that your blood sugar has remained relatively stable and that, assuming you didn't get stuck in rush-hour traffic on the way to work, your mood has, too.

So now you have a direct connection between your physiology and how you feel, which makes it easier to understand that eating an omelet instead of Pop-Tarts is not just "better for you" (whatever that means) but also makes you *feel* better. This emotional anchor point is more likely to encourage a change in behavior than a nutritionist's advice or a food log alone, and you used technology as a way to connect the dots between what you put into your mouth, its effect on your body, and the impact on your mood. So now that you have a strong cause-effect relationship and realize that changing your breakfast makes you feel better, you're more likely to kick your Pop-Tarts habit in favor of healthier choices.

70 Percent of the Time It Works Every Time

Fifty years ago, scientific studies usually involved just six to ten people, and the pool was composed of the researchers, their grad students, and their colleagues. Scientists recorded and published the individual data for everybody involved in the study. Then statistics started to become a bigger deal and the methodology changed. Suddenly, the individual responses were relegated to the background while averages came to the fore. This helped to conceal poor data and findings that appeared contradictory or inconclusive.

Looking solely at averages has obscured the reality that even things that have been rigorously tested in hundreds of experiments and have largely been shown to benefit most of the population don't work for everyone. Two cases in point are caffeine and creatine. Many believe that there's a consensus on the efficacy of these substances in improving performance. Few understand that a full 30 percent of people don't respond to what's considered an "average" amount of caffeine or the recommended creatine dose. You could well be one of them! If so, you'd need to play around with your intake to see how much you'd need to take to elicit a response—there are no tech-driven guidelines for you personally if you're in that group.

The advent of online research publications and aggregate sites promises to swing the pendulum back in the other direction. Now there are no longer the space constraints of a physical journal, which often limited scientists to using one graph of averages. Online, there's infinite room, so researchers can include as many graphical elements as they like. This heralds the welcome return of publishing each participant's individual data and responses to the control variable. In the coming years we're going to see many retractions of landmark studies that have formed the basis for entire fields and decades' worth of recommendations.

It's also inevitable that much of the research that supposedly demonstrates the effectiveness of fitness technology will be revealed to be exaggerated and grossly misleading. As we wait for this revolution to gather pace, we should reexamine what our technology is telling us and not take the science behind it at face value. We'd be better off fine-tuning our self-awareness and making adjustments based on what we're experiencing. As Carl Sagan said, science is a way of thinking much more than it is a body of knowledge. Data can be considered knowledge, but until this point in our history, most of what we thought we knew has been exposed as wrong (see: sugar is harmless; running lots of long, slow miles is the only way to become a good endurance athlete; and so on). So what makes us think that what we're doing right now is any different? Having more information can give us a useful starting point, but don't fall into the trap of believing that it proves anything beyond fallibility. Start with the data and then let your body, awareness of your environment, and your coach's experience guide you from there.

Do You Get High?

In *The Lego Movie*, the protagonist, Emmet, looks at a set of instructions each morning to see what he's meant to do. The final statement on the cover of this manual promises that if he just follows the rules, he will "always be happy." This is a cynical observation about our society's hyperoptimism but also an accurate one. We've elevated the pursuit of happiness above life and liberty, and when our epicurean lifestyle doesn't live up to expectations, we take pills to moderate our emotions because we think we're "depressed."

Fitness technology feeds into this need for constant happiness by rewarding us with an endless string of visual, auditory, and haptic encouragements and congratulations. And just like Emmet, we look to our devices to tell us what to do so we can achieve this perma-happy state.

What we've overlooked is that our physiology is constantly seeking a return to equilibrium, which means that for each high there needs to be a corresponding low to level us out. Frank Merritt believes that we've focused so much on stimulating our "happy hormones" that we've conveniently forgotten that others are meant to bring us down again. We might be pursuing constant happiness, but it's not natural or obtainable.

To rediscover emotional equilibrium and well-being, we need to first recognize the differences between happiness and joy. The former is a reaction to our surroundings that relies on an external stimulus, like a wearable vibrating when we hit a new personal best. Joy, on the other hand, is an intrinsic feeling that we often come to through trial and adversity. If we cease relying on a machine, the circumstances of our life, and other people's likes, retweets, and follows to provide happiness, we might be able to get closer to finding real joy. If you're unhappy, it might not be that you have too much suffering or adversity in your life but too little. Start seeking out experiences (preferably outdoors) that push you and make you feel uncomfortable (see chapter 9 for some suggestions).

In Pole Position

One of the keys to being a competent athlete and a fully functioning human being is developing the movement literacy needed to access all the basic movement archetypes—basic body positions, like a squat, lunge, and press—at any time and in any environment. That's one of the reasons I enjoy jiujitsu so much. Unlike some other martial arts that have rigid systems and require participants to memorize complex series of moves to earn their next belt, jiujitsu requires you to constantly improvise, whether you're standing or ground fighting. It has certain foundational principles, but these are applied fluidly, and no two grappling sessions or fights are ever the same. I also find practicing it to be a humbling experience, particularly when I'm being thrown around by current and former world champions!

The constant variation that you find in jiujitsu is similar to what I enjoy about surfing and stand-up paddleboarding, which put you in an environment that's always different and ever-evolving. There is no app, device, or piece of technology that can teach you what you need to excel—or even survive—in these activities. Immersion learning is the only way to

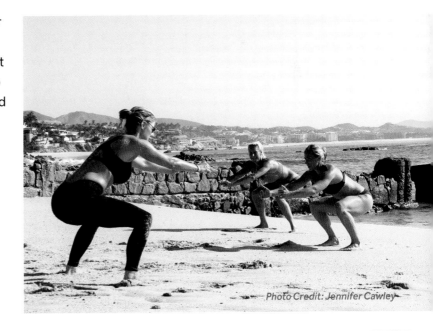

Photo Credit: Jennifer Cawley

become proficient, and doing so requires a time investment and complete mental, spiritual, and physical commitment.

Cues, Not Crutches

Earlier we looked at technology that coaches can use to improve your self-awareness and to reinforce teaching cues. There are also certain tools that you can use on your own to identify and self-correct mechanical, positional, and other issues. I'm not going to push any products on you in this book, but something I've found to be very helpful in my own training and that of my athletes is the Shoe Cue. This is essentially a piece of plastic with little knobs that you slip into the heel of each shoe. When you thud down onto those heels instead of landing softly on the balls of your feet and then lightly tapping your heels to the ground, you get immediate feedback—just enough of the "ah crap, there's a rock in my shoe" sensation to make you feel that you're not landing correctly.

We use the Shoe Cue during warm-ups to connect a mechanical fault that compromises performance and will cause injury if left unchecked to an exaggerated heel-striking sensation. Once my athletes instinctually identify the problem—heel striking—and then self-correct by landing on their forefoot instead, we're done with the Shoe Cue for the day. Now they can use their newly attuned self-awareness for the rest of the session.

Using coaching cues to improve self-awareness is backed up by the latest research. A recent study divided Olympic weight lifters into two groups. The first were told what they were doing wrong and how to correct it, such as, "The bar is coming out too far—keep it closer to you." The second group were told to exaggerate the thing they were doing wrong with a cue like "Push the bar further away from you," without being told what exactly they were doing incorrectly. Which group improved more?

Surprisingly, it was the second one. This is because by exaggerating the technique flaw, the athletes felt what they were doing wrong and were able to correct it.[121] Technology can be used to promote a similar increase in awareness. I have some of my athletes wear the Training Mask, a resistance breathing device, to teach better breathing patterns, and wearing a weight belt helps novices learn how to create abdominal pressure that protects their spine during squats. Digital technology that provides visual or audio feedback (such as beeps or buzzes) can help less-experienced athletes sense when they're doing something wrong, and once they're more cognizant of how they're moving, it can be removed.

The key here is that the athlete, coach, and technology are all involved, but the emphasis is on human learning and understanding. Relying on a gadget alone not only prevents you from developing self-awareness but can even result in harm if the device is inaccurate or gives faulty feedback.

Dream Bigger

We're often our own worst enemy. We set limits on what we believe we can do and fail to see beyond what already exists to what may be possible. We let fear of failure stop us from trying something new. But if we're able to shake off these self-imposed limitations, the sky is, literally, the limit.

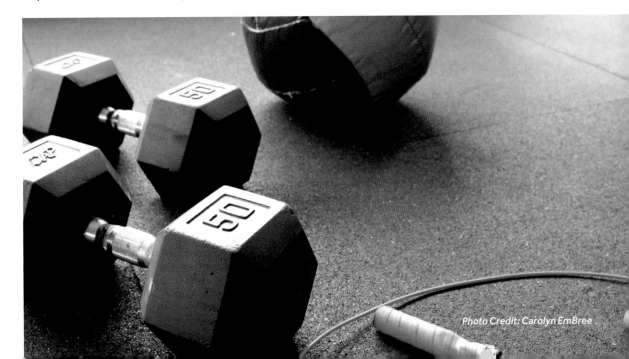

Photo Credit: Carolyn EmBree

From the Edge of Space

Many people find it useful to set defined goals—like running a sub-three-hour marathon or competing in an Ironman—and then work backwards to create smaller milestones toward those aims, so they can measure their progress over time. There's nothing inherently wrong with this, but there's always the risk that striving to achieve a certain time in a race, get on the podium, or reach a particular weight in your favorite lift can become restrictive. In one way, you're limiting yourself and trying to push your body just hard enough to reach this mark, and no more. Then, when you use your daily activity tracking and other kinds of monitoring to see where you're at and how close you are to where you want to be, the data can act as another barrier to the almost unlimited progress that I think we're all capable of.

One of the reasons I was so enthralled by Felix Baumgartner's 2012 jump from the edge of space was that he was redefining what was possible and showing that the term *impossible* is just, at its essence, an arbitrary and meaningless creation of our minds. When he made the leap into nothingness and managed to land safely—having had to stop a spin that could've killed him—I rejoiced not because he'd done it but because he'd set the bar at twenty-four miles into the stratosphere. And then, just a few months later, Google executive Alan Eustace went even higher. Felix's and Alan's stories illustrate that we've got to stop letting our own mediocre expectations and the trappings of technology limit us, because there truly are no limits except those we set for ourselves.

Another example of boundless progress in action is Kai Lenny, who is constantly moving between surfing, stand-up paddleboarding, kiteboarding, and other disciplines. Kai understands that one of the keys to being a true waterman is to believe that potential is infinite if you just remain open to any and all possibilities and take the time to appreciate whatever experiences may bring your way. This is why you shouldn't be limited by your own numerical goals or those provided by your wearable. Dream bigger than that and then, like Kai, go out and make that dream reality.

The Master Tinkerer

Kai's boundary-breaking in water sports is rooted in the progressive thinking of those who came before him. Many giant leaps in what is believed to be possible can be attributed to Laird Hamilton, whose experimentation created whole new ways to ride waves, like tow-in surfing, foiling, and stand-up paddleboarding. Here's what Laird said about his innovations.

I needed to improve my board control and balance in the summer to prepare for the winter storms, but there's no surf in Hawaii in the summer. I also wanted to take my kids out with me, so we began riding these bigger boards together. I saw benefits of manipulating these longer boards and then decided I didn't want to have to lie down to paddle into each wave. So I made this paddle and suddenly I could go out in flat conditions or small waves. Then I wanted to ride big waves and paddle across channels. All of a sudden you're catching more waves so you become better quicker. With tow surfing and foiling, we couldn't ride certain waves because of the surface conditions, so we used technology to solve that problem. If you've been doing something for fifty years you can get complacent or bored, so for me that's also been a driver of innovation. I've created things that've inspired me.[122]

James Dyson's 5,127 Tries

I chose "Unscared" as the handle for my social-media accounts and the tattoo on my hands not because I'm never afraid of anything but rather because I'm not too intimidated to try almost anything. This is one of the reasons that I'm constantly experimenting on myself to see what works, what doesn't, and what lessons I can learn along the way. Then I try to pass those on to others.

It took British inventor James Dyson 5,127 tries to perfect his bagless cyclone vacuum cleaner. Nobody had come close to creating such a revolutionary design, so he had to teach himself as he went along. This true autodidact could've quit many, many times. But he had a vision of what he wanted to create and was willing to spend five years and every penny he had to make it become a reality.

Like Dyson, we need to have big ideas, ignore those who think we're crazy for pursuing them, and just make them happen. Maybe that's something big, like summiting all the 14ers (peaks higher than 14,000 feet) in Colorado, or perhaps it's just a challenge that's intimidating for you, such as learning to swim. If you can use a device to help motivate you, track your progress, and share updates with friends, then go ahead and use one. But realize that lasting motivation doesn't come from a flashing display. If you're going to forge ahead and achieve a significant life goal, the desire has to be kindled inside you.

Ready, Set, Go

Thousands of years ago, hunter-gatherers didn't insist on doing ten minutes on a bike or rowing machine, spending twenty minutes on calisthenics, and then downing an energy drink or pre-workout amino shot before chasing their prey. They just did it. In today's corporate, money-driven culture, we've been swindled into thinking that if we don't check all

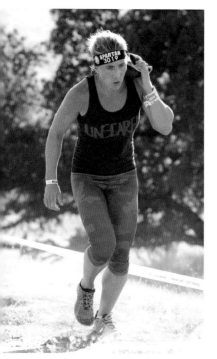

Photo Credit: Spartan Race, Inc.

these boxes, we're going to have a poor-quality workout or get hurt. We also get so comfortable in a highly regimented gym setting that we avoid the dynamic unpredictability of a fun activity like pickup basketball, rec league soccer, or a game of touch football, which would give us the chance to express the physical qualities we've been developing for so long in the weight room. Then we try to further limit the risk of failure, subpar performance, or even getting shown up by imprisoning ourselves indoors.

What we need to do is learn how to achieve a constant state of readiness and preparedness that enables us to mimic our ancestors and go from stationary to full speed, like Usain Bolt out of the starting blocks (okay, maybe not *quite* that fast, but you get my point). Some of the few people I know who are in such a ready state all the time are special operators in the Marines and Navy SEALs. Their training prepares them to respond to crises anywhere in the world on virtually no notice, and when they do deploy, they do so quickly, efficiently, and ruthlessly.

For those of us who aren't rushing to our nearest recruiting office to join these warriors in the field, we should try to keep ourselves sharp with a broad range of activities that continually challenge us in new ways. Think you're too old to ski or snowboard? Take some lessons this winter. Always wanted to skateboard? Buy one for yourself as well as your kid on their birthday and go scrape your elbows and knees together.

We need to remember that we learn from failing and getting hurt, not from eliminating risk (which isn't possible, by the way) and deifying safety. If you're hesitant to try something new, think about what's really stopping you. Is it truly time or lack of gear or money, as you might initially claim? It's more likely an ego issue: you're scared of looking like a newbie or being embarrassed. Drill down to find your mental roadblock and then insist on going over, around, or through it.

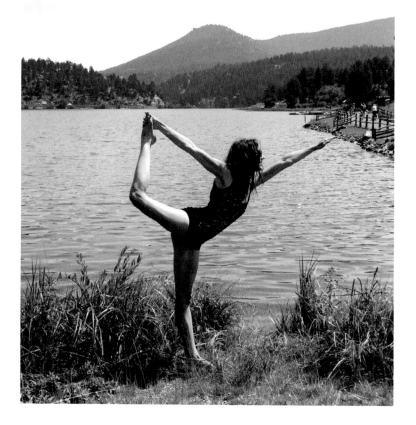

Make It Fun

I take training and movement seriously, but I never lose sight of the fact that in the end, it's supposed to be fun. Being active is something that should be pleasurable—but when we become focused on the numbers our devices tell us and getting the latest and greatest equipment, it sucks the joy out of practice.

Ending the Gear Arms Race

If you live in a mountain town, you've almost certainly seen a suburbanite show up on your favorite trail with his $300 sunglasses, $750 technical hardshell, and $400 custom hiking boots. The same is true at the beach, where total beginners will nonchalantly take a $3,000 carbon paddleboard out into the surf and then get beaten down in the first big set of the day. The phrase "All the gear and no idea" springs to mind.

Yet such people are a microcosm of the gear arms race that's intensifying in just about every sport and activity.

In cycling, it's the weight of your bike that seems to be the biggest issue for bragging rights. And once you've got the handmade $7,000 frame, then it's the minutiae of brakes, helmets, and the rest that keeps people forking over their hard-earned cash at their local bike shop. In our materialist society, we can buy just about anything we want on credit, and what we want is the lightest, the fastest, and the best-looking sports gear available. Keeping up with the Joneses is no longer about how big your house is or what car you drive but what gizmos you store in your garage and unload from your car.

This is good news for bike and surf shops, big-box stores like REI, and online behemoths such as Backcountry. But it's bad news for the sports themselves, which have lost the vibe of bohemian sixties surf culture, the dirtbag ethos cultivated in places like Yellowstone in the seventies, and the closeness of the tight-knit fell running fraternity in the UK during the eighties. Turn up at a local race in just about any sport now and it's like going to the Outdoor Retailer show, with everyone showing off the latest shiny toys. This not only takes the focus off the community but also puts off the newcomers needed to keep sports thriving in the future. They start to feel priced out if they don't have a few grand to drop on the latest and supposedly greatest gear.

In addition, it's foolish to think that possessing cutting-edge equipment will provide a massive competitive advantage. Give John John Florence a crappy, entry-level surfboard and he'd still destroy a beginner on a custom board. Put Scott Jurek in a pair of cheap tennis shoes and he's going to crush a recreational runner sporting $250 shoes.

Then there's the issue of identity. If your self-worth is dictated by the gear you've bought, you're leading a pretty small, unfulfilled life. This is not to say that you should never invest in quality, durable gear, but if it defines you and becomes more important than the activity you're using all this stuff for, then you might want to reexamine your priorities.

For Lenny Wiersma, it took a surf trip to Costa Rica to get a fresh perspective:

> I went with some friends who had these expensive boards, and if any of the Americans there got a ding in their board they'd say, "Well, I guess I'll have to buy a new one when I get home." Contrast that with these local teenagers who were riding these giant, clunky boards that looked like they were forty years old. In terms of skill level, they were just crushing all of us. Nobody in Newport Beach would even think of paddling out with a board like that and, if they did, it'd be useless because they're used to this light, maneuverable one. This reminded me that it's you that determines your performance, not the latest gear. Just use what you have available.[123]

Why So Serious?

When did all the enjoyment drain out of our physical practices? I'd argue that it was when we became obsessed with trying to quantify every minute detail. Perhaps this is related to how nuts we are for numbers in the sports we watch, wanting to know every baseball player's RBI, every basketball player's field goal percentage, and every quarterback's accuracy rating. Some people might enjoy the math part of examining all those statistics, but to me it takes the pleasure out of sports.

The same is true of the activities we participate in. Once you start using gadgets to record and quantify your performance, those stats can easily become the focal point. This not only is distracting but also robs you of the full experience that you can only have when you're totally focused on and committed to something that you love doing. Duke University professor Jordan Etkin wrote in a paper entitled "The Hidden Cost of Personal Quantification," "Let's say you like walking for fun. It's a relaxing, enjoyable activity, and you don't really have any other reason to do it. You just like it. When you start to track behaviors like that, it basically provides an external incentive for engaging in those other fun activities. And so you start to think more about how much you're doing, rather than just focusing on the enjoyment of the activity. It takes something that's fun and makes it more like work."[124]

If it's gotten to the point that your favorite sport feels like a chore or burden, whether that's because you've allowed a technology takeover or for any other reason, why the heck are you still doing it? Go find something new and fresh and see if it can reinvigorate you. Then come back to the original pursuit without any tech attached and see if you can learn to enjoy it again for its own sake.

Finding Equilibrium

Laird Hamilton is one of the most balanced people I know. When I asked him how being outside most of the day every day helps him maintain this, he said:

If you took someone who's indoors a lot of the time and got them into a routine of being outdoors more, their body chemistry and all of their functions would completely change. On a consciousness level, it would bring a kind of equilibrium.

I have a friend who's a famous basketball player, and I often tell him that when you're in a giant building with fifty thousand people screaming that they either love or hate you it's going to take a toll. The more you're in that kind of setting, the more you'd better go out and find a big tree somewhere and sit under it alone to counteract all of that other stuff. It's like a battery—you have the negative pull and the positive one. We have an indoor and outdoor pull. If everything's indoors, then there's going to be an imbalance in our battery. To create that balance, you need be exposed to the outdoors. We're from nature, we are nature. It is us and we are it.[125]

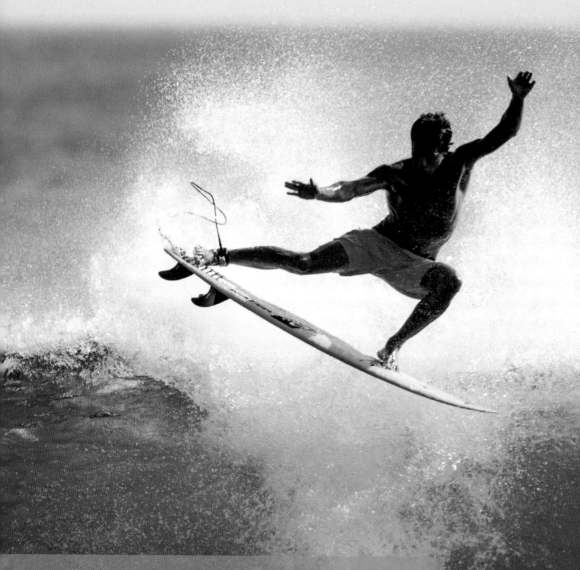

The Circle is almost complete, and Mae, you have to believe that this will be bad for you, for me, for humanity.

—Dave Eggers, The Circle

Photo Credit: Tom Servais

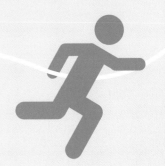

CHAPTER 9
PULL THE PLUG

In previous chapters we've looked at the history, philosophy, and psychology of an always-connected, technology-addicted lifestyle. I've shared cautionary tales, anecdotes, and before-and-after examples of fitness technology gone wrong, both from my own life and from more than fifteen years' experience of coaching athletes at every level. And we've looked at some practical ways in which you can use technology to enhance your self-awareness, retune your senses, and reconnect to your instincts. In addition, we've compared and contrasted a limited, constrained, device-dependent indoor existence with the boundless, explorative, self-reliant opportunities that fully immersing ourselves in nature offers.

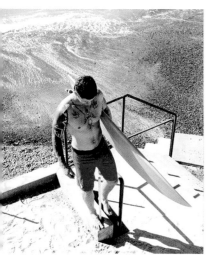

Photo Credit: Athletic Recon

Now that we've given you an ingredients list, it's time to share the recipe. To change your life and break out of the technology Matrix that many of us have been imprisoned in for far too long, you need to forgo technology algorithms for self-discovery, experimentation, and learning. A big part of the solution is in the very title and concept of this book: unplug more often, use technology as a learning aid instead of a taskmaster, and reengage with yourself, other people, and the natural world around you. But we'd be omitting something if we didn't leave you with some practical takeaways as well. So we brought in two of our good friends to help: Tim Ferriss and Steven Kotler.

Tim Ferriss's Top Ten Tips

In *The 4-Hour Body,* one of his *New York Times* best-selling books, Tim Ferriss reveals that he has recorded every workout since he was eighteen, taken over one thousand blood tests, and "spent more than $250,000 on testing and tweaking" in an effort to optimize his health, fitness, and wellness.[126] He has also interviewed many of the world's leading exercise scientists, performance specialists, and nutritionists; trained with renowned coaches, and studied a broad range of philosophical disciplines. So if anyone is qualified to dispense advice on this book's central themes, it's Tim. While I was, fittingly, walking up an Oregon mountain on a snowy afternoon in January 2017, Tim gave me his top ten tips for using fitness technology more effectively, enhancing your self-awareness, practicing presentness, and much more.

Determine in advance how much ability and time you have to interpret data, before you gather spreadsheet after spreadsheet's worth of data. When I've come to the wrong conclusion it's generally because I've collected more data than could be parsed effectively.

Decide what you're going to do with all this information by asking yourself the "three whys," each building on the previous answer. So if, for example, you're a cyclist who's going to track your heart rate, ask yourself:

Why am I going to track my heart rate?

Because I want to improve my lactate threshold.

Why do I want to improve my lactate threshold?

So I can maintain high power output longer.

Why will this help me?

Because usually I can't keep up with the pack in a race.

Ask these "whys" regularly. If you can answer all three, then you're getting somewhere. But if you can't get past the first one, then what you're doing is akin to managing symptoms instead of curing a disease. Terrible doctors treat symptoms, good doctors treat diseases, and great doctors treat people holistically. You can look at that from a data perspective as well. People who become slaves to their metrics without really thinking about the consequences of or intentions behind the data can end up chasing a number that, in isolation, means very little. At worst it can be counterproductive or even damaging, as when people chase a certain body fat percentage, assuming that lower is always better. That's simply not the case in many instances.

Change only one variable at a time so you don't mistake correlation for causation. If you've tried four new things at once, try to identify which one has the most plausibly explainable mechanism to create the positive change. Or try to isolate what actually was the causal factor by removing variables one at a time and seeing if the problem comes back.

Choose the right vehicle for your goals. If you have a purely recreational priority, ask yourself, "How much do I enjoy this?" Maybe you don't want to do high-intensity interval training. Instead, you want to have a leisurely game of tennis with a childhood friend for an hour, three times a week. That's totally fine.

If your priority is pure performance, ask yourself, "How much does this improve me?" I prefer to have a clear goal, whether that's optimizing for maximal strength, relative strength, or some type of metabolic conditioning that can be measured. Sometimes I'm working toward something that is less physical, like a book launch, and I'm in a holding pattern with my workouts. I'm very judicious and strategic about where I apply tracking.

Write your emotional responses to experiences in a journal to improve your self-awareness. You could use a physical notebook or an app like Five Minute Journal or Morning Pages. Journaling daily gives you a kind of semantic, instinctual feedback that type A personalities like me learn to mute subconsciously. We prefer to live through goals and spreadsheets and not feelings, which can be a handicap for life.

That's why I find it valuable to write about things that happened in my day and how I felt about them. I don't necessarily mean writing "I was angry" or "I was impatient" but rather noticing the physical feeling. What was your actual kinesthetic experience when someone said something, you were waiting for something, or you were doing a certain activity?

Another way to increase your awareness is to engage in some type of partner or group exercise that requires physical contact. For me, that's AcroYoga and jiujitsu. But it could be any combat sport, dance, or any number of other activities. Look at chimpanzees and you'll see they're in constant contact with each other. I think that is the medicine for a lot of what ails us: be more animal-like and less human-like, however you have constructed that to be different from other species.

Do different types of workouts for different purposes. For me, it's all about separating exercise and physical recreation with others. I have my "bitter medicine" sessions, which may involve heavy dead lifts with long rest intervals in between, during which I'm writing down what I'm doing and listening to music. I have other workouts that are slow-cadence weight lifting of some type or another, where I'm doing five to ten seconds up, five to ten seconds down. Both types of sessions are exercise, pure and simple. There's no recreational component intended, designed, or wanted.

Then I have days when I am playing with other people, such as in partner acrobatics. It's very much playful while simultaneously involving very difficult moves: maneuvering a partner, manipulating them with your feet, spinning them around. It's very focused on kinesthetic awareness and spatial awareness. When you are doing that well, there's nothing else you can think of and you're interacting with and responding to someone else. It's the same in jiujitsu, where there's an immediate penalty for any type of distraction or daydreaming. You'll get arm-barred or choked. There's incentive, punishment, and reward. You don't want to get choked again, so you change your behavior and learn to focus.

Start thinking about technology as a tool that you use for solving a problem. It's very easy for us to consider technology to be only something with a digital readout or something that is cutting-edge. But in nature, it's as simple as a stick that a

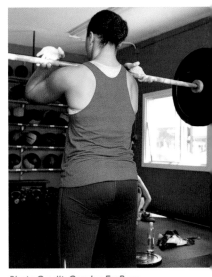

Photo Credit: Carolyn EmBree

chimpanzee pokes into an anthill. The most effective piece of fitness technology I've ever used is a notebook and pen to record my workouts. I'll then take photographs of each page using Evernote, so that I can search them for terms or dates or workouts.

After an ACL sprain, I wanted to get back into shape and focus on some combination of maximal and relative strength. I looked back at my notes and found an eight-week period from 1996 when I was focused very heavily on squats, dead lifts, and close-grip bench presses. If I knew I was applying a proper stimulus but wasn't improving in performance, then I'd just add more rest days. For each new workout, I'd put the number of days since I'd done the same workout. In doing so, I was able to identify the proper stimulus for my recovery abilities.

Now, after the ACL sprain, it's just plug and play. I'm taking that exact same recipe from 1996 and applying it, and I've made a huge amount of progress. I've lost around ten pounds of body fat and increased my strength dramatically—and that's just in the first, say, three to four weeks of training. I had that plan available because I'd taken the time to record my workouts properly.

Take time for daily present-state awareness training. You have to operate in the past, present, and future to be a fully functional human, but I've recognized that driven, type A personalities like me are very future-focused. We're very good at setting and achieving objectives, but if you never enjoy the process, if you can never celebrate the small wins, you're never going to be able to appreciate and celebrate the big wins, either. If that's the case, what's the point of setting all these goals in the first place? As Lao Tzu said, "If you are depressed, you are living in the past. If you are anxious, you are living in the future. If you are at peace, you are living in the present."

I've found meditation helpful in making me more aware of my present thoughts and state. Simultaneously you're training yourself to sit and do nothing, which allows you to appreciate when you have to do anything. The best example of this comes from the book *The Miracle of Mindfulness*, in which Thich Nhat Hanh writes about the mind-set most of us would be in if we decided to reward ourselves with a cup of tea after we finished doing the dishes:

> If, while washing the dishes, we think only of the cup of tea that awaits us, thus hurrying to get the dishes out of the way as if they were a nuisance, then we are not washing the dishes to wash the dishes. What's more, we are not alive during the time we are washing the dishes. In fact, we are completely incapable of realizing the miracle of life while standing at the sink. If we can't wash the dishes, the chances are we won't be able to drink our tea either. While drinking the cup of tea, we will only be thinking of other things, barely aware of the cup in our hands. Thus we are sucked way into the future and we are incapable of actually living one minute of life.[127]

Mindfulness helps you not only to focus on the now but also to be less reactive. For me, it helps mitigate some of my impulses to impatience or anger because I recognize the onset symptoms before they completely sabotage my thought process or boil over into some interpersonal interaction where everything goes south quickly. Consistency is more important than duration. Meditating every day for ten minutes over a ten-day period is much more impactful for me than if I meditate for twenty minutes every other day over a five-day period.

Get out and enjoy nature for its own sake without any technology. I think being outside is our natural state, and the more we override it or deny our natural inclinations, the more difficult life tends to be. I feel like we should exercise traits or abilities that we've made many evolutionary trade-offs to develop. When I do that, I am a calmer, happier, more effective human being.

Don't use as much technology as you can handle. Use the least amount necessary.

Steven Kotler's Guide to Focusing on Flow

In his landmark book *The Rise of Superman,* Steven Kotler explores how the world's best extreme-sports athletes have torn up the rule and record books, broken through boundaries, and propelled their disciplines to heights that were unimaginable even ten years ago by hacking flow: the elevated consciousness that not only propels action-sports stars into the physical and cognitive stratosphere but also has the potential to launch you far beyond your perceived limitations. In addition, Kotler has worked with top entrepreneurs like his *Abundance* coauthor Peter Diamandis, elite special forces groups, and tech innovators like Elon Musk in a wide-ranging study of peak states, which you can read more about in his outstanding book *Stealing Fire.* Kotler also collaborates with some of the brightest minds in the scientific, athletic, and artistic communities as he and his colleagues at the Flow Genome Project dive deeper into how we can map, trigger, and prolong flow. Here are some of Kotler's top tips for jump-starting your personal performance and well-being revolution and changing how you view the world for the better.

Spend less time in your office to get more done. I told somebody the other day that I spend a minimum of three and a half months of the year outside, between hiking, walking my dogs, skiing, mountain biking, and surfing. They were just flabbergasted and asked, "But how do you work?" I replied, "That's how I work." That's how I can run two companies and write a book every year and a half and do everything else I do. The more flow I get outside, the more flow I bring into my office in the morning when I'm writing. The more flow you have, the more flow you can get. It's a focusing skill that involves carving neural pathways. In McKinsey's ten-year study, top executives reported being 500 percent more productive in flow. We know from the DARPA studies that learning goes up 470 percent in flow. Motivation goes through the freaking roof, and we also know that creativity, accelerated learning, and creative problem-solving spike.

Set aside the tech if you want to find flow. When I work with skiers, I tell them to focus on the feeling of speed and fluidity, not a specific metric. If I'm stopping to look at what my heart rate monitor is telling me, it's not doing me any good. Now, if I'm recording my heart rate over the course of a day and can quickly push a certain thing on my watch while I'm on a chairlift between runs to see if I'm in zone A, B, C, or D, and I can use the data to steer back toward where I want to be? Interesting. But in the moment, I think technology is going to pull you out of flow. It's going to break the uninterrupted concentration you need.

Get outside to clear your mind and boost your mood. Twenty-first-century "normal," neurobiologically speaking, is tired, wired, and chronically stressed. What does it look like in the body? Hyperactivity in the prefrontal cortex, a steady drip-drip-drip of stress hormones like cortisol and norepinephrine, and brain waves in the high beta range, which is essentially agitated. You should have lower beta waves if you and I were just having a conversation, but in the twenty-first century, most of us are actually in the high beta range most of the time. That's now normal.

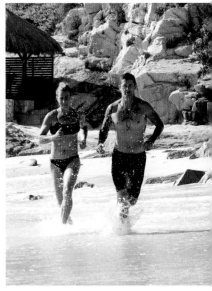

Photo Credit: Jennifer Cawley

That's insane. Those reactions were meant to show up when we had a fight-or-flight response when we encountered a saber-toothed tiger and had to run. They were not meant to be daily life. How do we know? Well, about one in six Americans are currently on antidepressants and antianxiety meds and 8 percent or more have PTSD.[128]

We've got fifty years of eco-psychology that tells us being in nature is fundamentally healing. We know a twenty-minute walk in the woods outperforms every SSRI on the market. We are wired to be in nature, and when we cut ourselves off from that, we're cutting ourselves off evolutionarily from our source. Without access to nature and the opportunity to throw myself down mountains at high speed, I can't do anything else. I can't write. I'm a lousy husband. I'm a lousy friend. All the things that are important to me don't happen.

Trade your treadmill for the trail. Every morning I walk my dogs through the backcountry for about forty-five minutes to an hour. There's a little bit of a walking path that goes for about twenty minutes and then I get into the real raw country. I know that, whatever my brain was doing beforehand, every day by the time I get to the end of that, my prefrontal cortex is shut down and it's quiet upstairs. We know through Arne Dietrich's work at Georgia Tech that there's such a thing as exercise-induced transient hypofrontality—which means that exercise can slow down your brain's prefrontal cortex, which governs cognitive functions, will, and sense of self. But I can't get there on a treadmill, and I have not found a way to get there any other way indoors. I've never once run myself into exercise-induced transient hypofrontality on my treadmill, even if I've exhausted myself until I can't move. Yet I can access that state almost every time I'm outdoors.

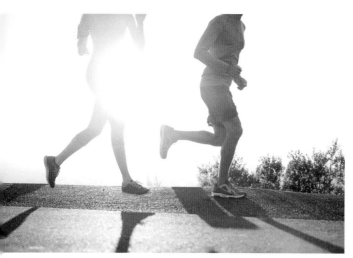

To save our planet, start seeing nature. There's fifty years of data coming out of psychology that says most people don't see the natural world, which is why our planet is having a giant environmental crisis. This is especially true in our modern lives, in which more and more of our world is packaged or on devices for us. Why are we in the middle of a giant biodiversity crisis? Most people don't see trees. They don't see animals. They don't even understand that they're part of the natural world around them because they don't spend enough time interacting with it. The problem is one of what they call ecological perception, and we're blind to it. The only way to really shift our perspective is to spend more time in nature. There's no other way. Fundamentally, if we're going to save our planet, we have to start seeing the actual planet.

The newest path to peak performance is the oldest one. A lot of the measurement technology is trying to hack the body. Unless you're an elite athlete who's in the top 5 percent and trying to get into the top 1 percent, I don't know what you're measuring. I can understand the value of certain baselines, but once you've achieved a certain level of fitness, the biggest bang for your buck is going to be in hacking your brain, not your body.

That essentially means hacking flow. The easiest way I know to do that is to send you outside. It's just faster, a shorter distance from A to B. We started thinking we were superior to nature and separated ourselves from it four hundred years ago, when we began believing that "I think, therefore I am" and privileged the rational mind above everything else.

Now we've come to the end of our psychological tether. We've done what we can do with technology, and it's time for some new methodologies. The data seems pretty overwhelming to me that one of the newest methods— returning to nature—is actually one of the oldest ones. We evolved in a natural environment, so going back into the environment is one of the best and simplest solutions.

Be your best when you're at your worst. I believe that there are five kinds of grit [per University of Pennsylvania psychology professor and author of *Grit,* Angela Duckworth: Optimism + Confidence + Creativity = Resilience = Hardiness = (+/-)Grit], and if you're really interested in high performance, you've got to train all of them. One of the most important things is training to be at your best when you're at your worst, and you can't just develop that cognitively. You have to train it physically at the same time.

That's why when I'm preparing for my speeches, I recite them on hikes up a mountain. That way, I know if I show up to give a speech and I'm exhausted and I haven't slept for three days and I'm sick with a stomach virus, I can still deliver the speech because I can do it while hiking uphill. To train for being at your best when you're at your worst, you need to train when you're cold, wet, and far from home.

I also apply this when I'm skiing. Once I get to the end of the day and I'm freezing, starving, and exhausted on the ski hill, I coax two more rounds out of myself, every time. I say, "Okay, you're done. You're taxed. You owe me two runs no matter what, at full speed." That's how I train for adversity. I can do it while mountain biking, too. I don't know how to do it in an office. You need the natural world for that.

Stop quantifying, start playing. A lot of companies are selling things to help you get closer to flow. But the research hasn't been done, at all. Nothing. No single biomarker has ever been correlated with flow. We know it's not just one factor but rather a lot of things happening at the same time, and that it's different for each individual. All we have at the moment is a flow state questionnaire. Adam Gazzaley's lab at UCSF is probably closest to developing a biophysical device, but they're grappling with the question of what engagement really means and what the line is between engagement and flow. That's A.

B is that flow is really a playful state. It can be helpful to have clear goals, but the reason they're important is so you know what you're doing today and what you're going to do next so you don't have to think about it. Seeking flow through a biometric isn't going to work, and the main reason is that flow has what we call a "deep embodiment trigger": it requires engaging multiple senses at once and being deeply in your body. Flow also has a rich environment trigger: it needs lots of novelty, lots of complexity, and lots of unpredictability. That's what being playful in nature gives you. You're using your body and all your senses tend to be engaged. Unless you're running on a clear, manicured trail, your footing is variable. There's a lot of stuff going on, and there are a lot of flow triggers packed in there.

What works best to transition you through the four stages of flow—struggle, release, flow, and recovery—is low-grade physical activity. If you look at the research, it shows the positive effects Albert Einstein got from rowing in the middle of Lake Geneva. Long walks in nature. Working in the garden. It's low-grade, in-nature stuff that provides the very easiest way to turn off the prefrontal cortex.

Take up an extreme sport. I think the risk and creative expression inherent in action sports are more important than location, but most of them take place outside. Training risk and kinesthetic creativity simultaneously is essential. I think you should be training creativity in everything, but if you're not doing it with your body, you're missing out on what I believe is the richest, most meaningful experience on earth.

I get into the deepest flow states when I'm skiing, downhill mountain biking, or surfing. Those are the deepest non-ordinary states of consciousness, even including psychedelic states. Those take me where I need to go, and I have enough expertise in those sports to get into these deep flow states 90 percent of the time or more. Try different things and see what works for you.

Immerse yourself in the natural world. For example, go to a rainforest and stay long enough that you forget the regular world and you can actually start seeing the rainforest. Go have one of those experiences. I'm an animal guy, so if I'm not hurling myself down mountains at high speeds, I'm someplace where I can be in the wild with animals. If that isn't you, go anywhere that you can start to understand how nature works.

One of the most amazing things you can see once you're immersed in nature is how the natural world changes over time. You actually get to see the forces that built the planet play out. For example, I've walked the same five to seven stretches of backcountry for the past ten years. Along the way, I've gotten to see how weather changes geology and how radically that stuff can happen. If you want to better understand yourself and nature, you have to be in nature.

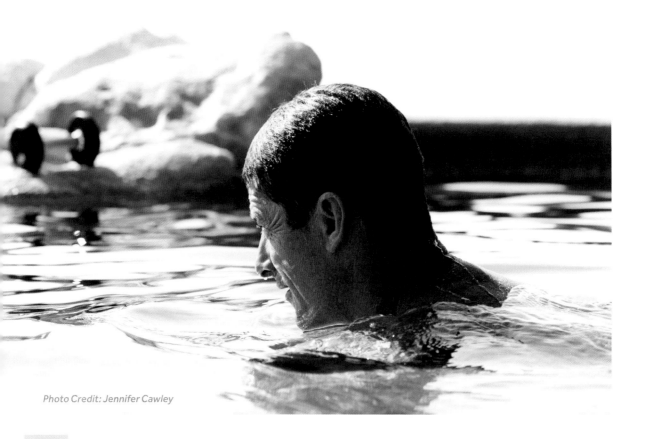

Photo Credit: Jennifer Cawley

The Principles of *Unplugged*

As we've covered so much ground in the previous eight chapters, I think it's time we recap some of the main points. However, keep in mind that since this is not a cookbook with 101 recipes or a dogmatic do-as-I-say rule book, you're going to have to interpret what I've presented to you and start your own self-experiment to see how you best can enhance your own health, fitness, and performance.

A large part of what I'm recommending to you is present in the title, *Unplugged*. As an individual who is designed to be self-reliant while remaining part of a society that has become too dependent on technology, too disconnected from its human essence, and too far removed from nature, you will, I firmly believe, reap many benefits by simply unplugging more often. If you can become more aware, retune your instincts, and get back in touch with your intuition, you'll become a happier, healthier human being. And the way to do this is not by outsourcing more of your decision-making to technology as part of an indoor lifestyle but by reclaiming responsibility for your wellness and resensitizing yourself in unfiltered experiences in the natural world. Here are the two key principles that can help you do just that.

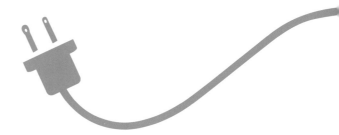

Don't Misuse Technology

If, after reading this book, you think you might be overusing or misusing technology, you're probably right. You should reduce your reliance on technology and change how you're wielding it if you use it to:

- Blunt your feedback from your environment and buffer bad form, such as with thick-soled shoes
- Deaden your senses, like cutting off your hearing by listening constantly to music or diminishing natural light exposure by always wearing sunglasses outdoors
- Reduce your physical activity to quantification, without paying any attention to the quality of your experiences
- Gather data that you don't know how to interpret
- Push yourself too hard, too often, so that your overall health suffers and you get injured regularly
- Substitute online interaction for real community
- Tell you what, how much, and when to eat, drink, or sleep
- Spend hours a day crunching numbers
- Replace the expertise of a coach
- Brag or boast about your achievements on social media sites
- Up the ante in the gear arms race or show off a status symbol

Use Technology Judiciously

Rather than going cold turkey on fitness technology, you can use it discerningly and in a deliberate, targeted way to:

- Give you early motivation to start moving more if you've been sedentary or are coming back from injury
- Connect how you feel and perform to your biology
- Enhance your ability to identify technique errors and then correct them
- Remind yourself to take movement breaks throughout the day
- Gain insight into a specific problem that is holding back your performance and is linked to a certain metric

- Guide your breathing until you become aware enough of your breath cycle to set the app aside
- Improve your understanding of a technique or topic, such as by watching videos or listening to podcasts
- Provide insights through mid- to long-term patterns that are visible in daily data collection
- Review data for specific sessions after your workouts, so the technology doesn't distract you during them
- Improve your safety through the use of SOS beacons, avalanche bags, and so on
- Find new running trails, bike paths, and other challenges through online communities

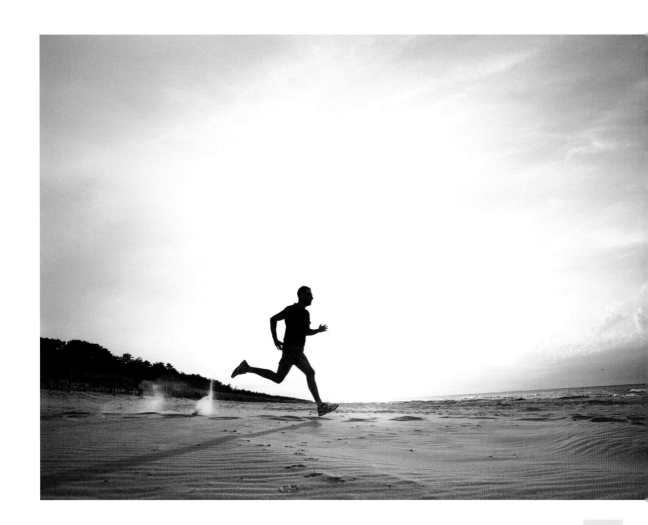

Tech to Consider

While I firmly believe in the importance of stepping away from tech and devices—see: the rest of this book—there are some tools that I've found to be particularly helpful or that merit further investigation. I'm not even coming close to saying that you need these to have a fruitful and fun practice, but they may be items to consider as a way of enhancing your training.

She's Electric

Since Kelly Starrett and I became friends more than a decade ago, I've used his movement and mobility techniques to greatly improve my performance and recovery, and introduced his system to all my athletes. Kelly's line of mobility tools plays an important role in my soft-tissue practice and are very effective by themselves. He and I have both realized that we can recover even faster when we add electrical muscle stimulation (EMS) into the mix. EMS works in a number of different ways, including resetting the nervous system, improving blood flow, and helping the body flush out the waste products that are produced during exercise. This is one technology I recommend wholeheartedly to all my athletes because I've used my Marc Pro device for years, have seen immediate and lasting benefits, and haven't experienced any side effects. If you want to improve recovery, ask your coach about going electric.

This isn't to say that EMS can't be misapplied. Some people can overuse it and get a false sense of recovery, or they're unable to function if their unit breaks or they have to travel without it. Using manual tools—like the MobilityWOD ones from Kelly Starrett—as well can help heighten your awareness of your range of motion and any restrictions you might have more effectively than electrical stimulation alone. Also, avoid blunting adaptation by doing too much EMS too soon after you exercise. It's best to incorporate this technology as just one tool in your recovery protocol.

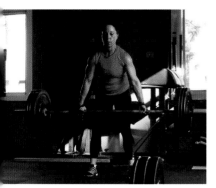

Photo Credit: Carolyn EmBree

Finding Flow

In his seminal book *The Rise of Superman*, Steven Kotler explores how getting into a fully focused, totally engaged flow state accelerates learning and cultivates progress. (Some of his top tips are in this chapter, starting on page 220.) He cites action sports athletes who find flow while outdoors, in thriving communities, and when engaged in activities that involve risk and danger. Some of the principles Kotler introduces for getting into a flow state preclude the use of technology, including eliminating distractions, focusing fully on what you're doing, and immersing yourself in an environment that's complex, unpredictable, and ever-changing. Simply put, you have to feel to flow.[129]

And yet one developing area of technology offers some promise in this area. We've looked at the benefits of using electrical stimulation for recovery, but what if you could also stimulate certain areas of your brain to put you in a flow state? That's what Dr. Daniel Chao, founder of Halo Neuroscience, is hoping to do through neuropriming. Neuropriming uses a small electrical current (which the makers swear is safe) to stimulate the motor cortex of the brain, which plays a big part in movement and the kinesthetic learning that comes with it.

Chao's company is introducing neuropriming to the masses with the Halo headphones, which you wear for a few minutes before you perform your activity of choice. According to the company's website, neurotechnology helped the military accelerate pilot and sniper training by 50 percent, while athletes training at Michael Johnson Performance's HQ increased explosiveness by 12 percent, versus 3 percent increases for the control group.[130] I haven't tested the Halo headphones and the field is still in its infancy, but it's fascinating from a coaching standpoint. If you could turn up primed and ready to learn every day, my job as a coach would be a lot easier and you'd get more out of each session. There might be some downside that we don't know about yet, so proceed cautiously if you decide to try neuropriming.

The *Unplugged* Road Map

Earlier in the book, we shared multiple examples of how you can use technology in a limited capacity to elevate feeling, identify problems, and correct them. The ability to do so varies according to your level of experience and the degree to which you've come to rely on technology. You might consider yourself to be an intermediate or even advanced athlete, but you might still be at a novice level when it comes to awareness of your body and how it's interacting with your environment. This doesn't mean you're any less of a human being; in fact, it only makes you more human. Awareness is not a fast-food restaurant drive-through; it takes serious time, and we believe we can help.

I think we'd be doing you a disservice if we didn't provide you with some concrete guidance at this point. That's why we've come up with the *Unplugged* program, which seeks to encapsulate some of the main principles in this book in an easily applicable protocol that you can start using, whether you're a pro athlete, weekend warrior, or anything in between. One of the key goals should be to improve your level of self-awareness and engagement as you progress, while simultaneously decreasing your dependence on technology. Although the *Unplugged* program covers only four weeks, use these four weeks to guide your next four, the following four, and so on, until you're ready for the next level.

Depending on what level you're at—novice, competitor, or pro—you'll need to utilize technology to a different extent as you work through the program in this chapter (or the personalized version of it that you come up with later).

The Conconi Test: Establishing a Baseline

To help establish some useful baselines that will provide guidance for the *Unplugged* program, you need to first take a modified version of the Conconi test. This assessment, which measures your anaerobic and aerobic threshold heart rates, is something I've worked on extensively with Florida A&M University exercise physiologist Dr. Brian Hickey. He has pioneered a ton of work on things a lot of people do not know about, and as well as being a mad scientist who is a ton of fun to talk with and learn from, he also holds more national titles than anyone I know.

The Conconi test looks for four stress responses. It works in a linear fashion, which means the stress response—heart rate increase—should also be linear. If we see a normal jump in your heart rate of five beats for two to three rounds and then there's an eight-beat jump, we know you just had a larger stress response and there's an issue that might need some ironing out, such as improving your pulmonary function. Here's how to warm up for and conduct the test:

Warm-Up

We recommend warming up on the machine and modality that you are going to test on, such as a rowing machine, Assault AirBike, or treadmill. If you have a resistance breathing device such as a Training Mask or Expand-A-Lung, we suggest using it throughout the whole warm-up to help better prepare your respiratory system. If you do not have such a device, that's okay—just proceed with the following warm-up to prep your system as best as possible.

> 3 minutes easy (40–50 percent effort)
> 5 rounds of 20 seconds on, 40 seconds easy (progress your 20-second efforts until the last one is at 90 percent)
> 1 minute easy
> 90 percent effort for 45 seconds (you should have something in the tank at the end, but do *not* use it)
> 5 minutes rest (try to get your heart rate back down to 99)
> Then administer the test

The Test

If you're fit and using an Assault AirBike, we suggest men start at 48 rpm, women start at 44–46 rpm (if you're under 5'6", we recommend 44 rpm, which has nothing to do with being female or your height but rather the setup of the bike). If you're unfit, men should begin at 44 rpm and women at 42 rpm. Increase rpm by two every minute, until you feel you can no longer continue or cannot maintain the rpm for more than five seconds.

Using equipment other than the Assault AirBike for the test? If you're fit and utilizing a machine that measures wattage (like the Concept2 erg or Ski Erg), we suggest men start at 180 watts and women at 150 watts. Increase the wattage by 20 every minute, until you can't continue or cannot maintain the wattage for more than five seconds. If you're unfit, men should start at 150 watts and women at 120. Then increase the wattage by 10 every minute, until you cannot continue or can't maintain wattage for more than five seconds.

If you're using a treadmill and are fit, both men and women should start at half-a-percent grade and 4.5 mph (7.2 kph) and

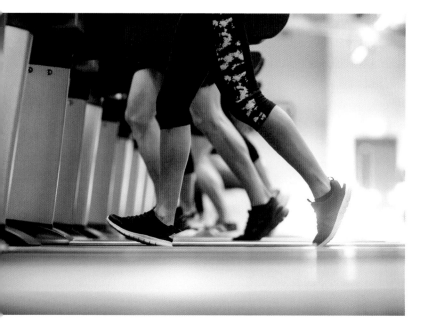

move up 0.5 mph (0.8 kph) every minute. If you're unfit, both men and women should start at zero percent grade, at a speed of 3.0 mph (4.8 kph), and move up 0.5 mph (0.8 kph) every minute, until you cannot continue.

For all tests, at the top of each minute, have a partner note your heart rate. It is important that you get the heart rate at the top (or end) of each minute (0:59, 1:59, 2:59, and so on).

Example: Fit Male, Assault AirBike

0:59: 48
1:59: 50
2:59: 52
3:59: 54
4:59: 56
5:59: 58
6:59: 60
7:59: 62
8:59: 64
9:59: 66
10:59: 68
11:59: 70

Note: You can use rpm, wattage, or pace with the same calculations.

Applying Testing Numbers to the *Unplugged* Program

Now you've obtained some baseline data that will guide each day of the *Unplugged* program, here's a little bit more context about the three levels and what you should be aiming for as you progress through each one. Try to objectively assess your ability level or, if you need help, ask a more experienced training partner or your coach. If you think you're between levels, drop down to the lower one, as it'd be more beneficial to get things right here than to go too far too soon at the higher level.

Novice: Obtain a fundamental understanding of how you feel as you progress physiologically, technically, and mechanically through levels of intensity, based on your movement patterns, joint angles, and physical abilities. You should always be striving for improvement and greater efficiency. To help you progress, you can spend a year self-experimenting to find the best path for you, using the *Unplugged* program as a guide but also trying new outdoor activities or challenging yourself to build on existing skills. In addition, go beyond this book in attending a reputable workshop and educating yourself with books, podcasts, blogs, and so on. You might also find it beneficial to start working with an experienced coach. If you don't have one or can't find one locally, we can help you out at Power Speed Endurance (powerspeedendurance.com).

In addition, you could use a mirror or camera and a live feedback technology app like Coach's Eye to capture and then watch your movement. Take note of key errors and how your body felt when you made them. Have a coach explain the gold standard for the movement and then use the app and mirror or camera to help achieve it. The combination of coaching and technology can help you in (1) identifying the error and physiological changes, (2) knowing what to do about it, and (3) recognizing if your adjustment actually fixes the dysfunction. It could be as easy as just slowing down! You can also use a heart rate monitor periodically to see if your perceived exertion correlates to actual physiological output.

Competitor: Strive to reach a competency level at which you can make the necessary adjustment when the technical error is pointed out or, more importantly, when you *feel* it. Use the same technology that a novice would at the end of each session or periodically during that work (such as a mirror, camera, app, and heart rate monitor). At this point, you should understand the feelings associated with physiological changes and movement enough to know what to do to make the change and whether or not that fixed the problem.

Pro: Use a coach or app occasionally to make sure that how you're feeling and how you're gauging your exertion and intensity matches up with the numbers. However, you don't truly own a movement or position until you can feel yourself making an error, identify the issue, and fix it independently. So work hard to master your technique, elevate your awareness of how you're going through each stage, and hone your ability to identify and self-correct problems. Also try to be more conscious of when you're undergoing physiological changes and how this impacts your breathing, posture, and technique/mechanics. It's okay for you or your coach to occasionally use technology to give you greater insight into what these changes are, how they should make you feel, and how you can best deal with them, but it should be an educational aid, not a daily crutch.

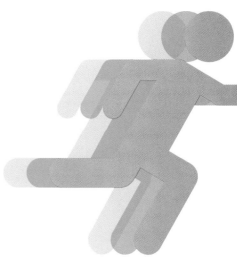

The Blueprint

To get you started on the road to a sustainable, healthy, and transformative movement practice that relies more on your instincts and interaction with your environment than it does on technology, I've combined the best of what I've learned in more than fifteen years of coaching into the following program. The first step is to accurately and honestly assess whether you fit into the novice, competitor, or pro category, outlined above. The second is to commit to consistent effort and self-discovery. This is merely a blueprint, so feel free to keep what works, discard what doesn't, and modify the program to suit your individual needs and progress. Now, let's get going.

Abbreviations

HR Heart rate

LI Long interval

SI Short interval

LAE Low intensity aerobic work

TT Tempo or time trial

Stage	Watts (Work)	HR	Deflection
1	130	120	
2	145	135	15
3	160	138	3
4	175	144	6
5	190	148	4
6	205	152	4
7	220	156	4
8	235	163	7
9	250	165	2
10	265	171	6
11	280	176	5
12	295	181	5

LAE

1

2

3

Your **HR** should not exceed these numbers until you can feel the changes that inevitably occur at a higher **HR**.

Endurance **TT**	< 144
LI	< 163
SI	< 171
LAE	< 135

NOVICE

WORK AND REST	WHEN TO STOP
SI will consist of < 3:00 efforts where maximal **HR** cannot exceed your **SI** number. Start by resting for 2:00 between each **SI** for the first few weeks, until you know you've made adaptations.	1. Pain 2. Technical/mechanical changes 3. **HR** increases past **SI** number 4. Times get slower each round by more than 5 seconds
LI will consist of work between 3:00 and 7:00 where maximal **HR** cannot exceed your **LI** number. Start by resting for 3:00 between each **LI** for the first few sessions, until you know you've made adaptations.	1. Pain 2. Technical/mechanical changes 3. **HR** increases past **LI** number 4. Times get slower each round by more than 8 seconds
Endurance (**TT** work in Power Speed Endurance) will consist of work for > 20 minutes and you must keep your **HR** under your Endurance (1) **HR** target.	1. Pain 2. Technical/mechanical changes 3. Slow down or walk if **HR** increases past endurance number
LAE will be work done outside like doing your sport at a leisurely pace (paddling, cycling, etc.) or doing yard work, hiking, gardening, etc, and your **HR** cannot exceed the **LAE** mark.	1. Pain 2. Technical/mechanical changes 3. If **HR** increases past **LAE**, stop work until it drops below that number

It's your job to correlate the feeling of these numbers and take notes to make sense of them. Although you will be glued to your **HR** monitor for a few sessions, the idea is to unglue so you can feel what certain exertion levels feel like. All the numbers will change as your physiology progresses, so calibrating this awareness is crucial.

	WEEK 1	WEEK 2	WEEK 3	WEEK 4
Day 1 (SI)	3–5 sets	3–5 sets	4–6 sets	4–6 sets
Day 2 (LI)	2–4 sets	2–4 sets	3–5 sets	3–5 sets
Day 3 (TT/Endurance)	20 min	20–30 min	30–45 min	30–45 min
LAE (Yard work, gardening, shoveling, slow paddling, cycling, etc)	30–90 min	40–110 min	60–120 min	60–120 min

NOVICE

COMPETITOR

WORK AND REST	WHEN TO STOP
SI will consist of < 3:00 efforts where maximal **HR** cannot exceed your **SI** number. Start by resting for 2:00 between each **SI** for the first week, then drop 15 seconds off the rest each week thereafter. DO NOT look at **HR** during work, only at the end of the working interval so that you can make adjustments and feel more of what is going on.	1. Pain 2. Technical/mechanical changes 3. You cannot keep **HR** below **SI** number at end of work 4. Times get slower each round by more than 4 seconds
LI will consist of work between 3:00 and 7:00 where maximal **HR** cannot exceed your **LI** number. Start by resting for 3:00 for the first week, then drop 15 seconds off of the rest each week thereafter. DO NOT look at **HR** during work, only at the end of the working interval so that you can make adjustments and feel more of what is going on.	1. Pain 2. Technical/mechanical changes 3. You cannot keep **HR** below **LI** number at end of work 4. Times get slower each round by more than 6 seconds
Endurance (**TT** work in Power Speed Endurance) will consist of work > 20 minutes and you should try to keep **HR** under your Endurance (1) **HR**. Only look at your **HR** every 5 to 10 minutes to check where you are at and to make any corrections. The goal is to get to the point where you know and feel how much exertion it takes to stay at this intensity level and only need to recheck your **HR** occasionally for calibration.	1. Pain 2. Technical/mechanical changes 3. Slow down or walk if **HR** increases past Endurance number
LAE will be work done outside, like doing your sport (cycling, paddling, etc.) at a leisurely pace, or doing yard work, hiking, gardening, etc. Your **HR** cannot exceed the **LAE** mark. DO NOT check your **HR** until you're done. That way you can start to feel more of what's going on, and this intensity level allows for more mistakes than others that are more demanding.	1. Pain 2. Technical/mechanical changes

It's your job to correlate the feeling of all these numbers and take notes to make sense of them. After a couple of weeks, you should not be glued to your **HR** monitor as much as you were initially. The idea is for you to become conscious of how much exertion is needed and what this feels like. Your numbers will change, but the perceived exertion should be the same. Are you seeing/feeling this? If not, use your **HR** monitor to recalibrate, then test again without looking at it until after a session.

	WEEK 1	WEEK 2	WEEK 3	WEEK 4
Day 1 (SI)	4–6 sets	4–6 sets	5–7 sets	5–7 sets
Day 2 (LI)	3–5 sets	3–5 sets	4–6 sets	4–6 sets
Day 3 (TT/Endurance)	30–45 min	40–60 min	45–80 min	45–80 min
LAE (Chores, yard work, gardening, shoveling, etc.)	60–90 min	60–120 min	60–120 min	60–120 min

COMPETITOR

PRO

WORK AND REST	WHEN TO STOP
SI will consist of < 3:00 efforts, where maximal **HR** cannot exceed your **SI** number. Start by resting for 2:00 between each **SI** interval for the first week, then drop 15 seconds off the rest each week thereafter. DO NOT look at **HR** during the entire workout. Just record it, and then go back and see if you were able to connect your feelings with the numbers.	1. Pain 2. Technical/mechanical changes 3. Times get slower each round by more than 4 seconds
LI will consist of work between 3:00 and 7:00 where maximal **HR** cannot exceed your **LI** number. Start by resting for 3:00 for the first week, then drop 15 seconds off of the rest each week thereafter. DO NOT look at **HR** during entire workout. Just record it and then go back and see if you were able to connect your feelings with the numbers.	1. Pain 2. Technical/mechanical changes 3. Times get slower each round by more than 6 seconds
Endurance (**TT** work in Power Speed Endurance) will consist of work > 20 minutes and you want to keep **HR** under your Endurance (1) **HR** target by feeling only! DO NOT look at **HR** during the entire workout. Just record the workout, then go back and see if you were able to connect your feelings with the numbers.	1. Pain 2. Technical/mechanical changes
LAE will be work done outside, like performing your sport (cycling, paddling, etc.) at a leisurely pace or doing chores, (farming, gardening, etc.). Your **HR** cannot exceed the **LAE** mark. DO NOT check your **HR** until you're done. That way you can start to feel more of what's going on, and this intensity level allows for more mistakes than others that are more demanding.	1. Pain 2. Technical/mechanical changes

It's your job to correlate the feeling of all these numbers and take notes to make sense of them. After a couple of weeks, you should not be glued to your **HR** monitor as much as you were initially. The idea is to become conscious of how much exertion is needed and what this feels like. Your numbers will change, but the perceived exertion should be the same. Are you seeing/feeling this? If not, use your **HR** monitor to recalibrate, then test again without looking at it until after a session.

	WEEK 1	WEEK 2	WEEK 3	WEEK 4
Day 1 (SI)	5–8 sets	5–8 sets	6–8 sets	6–8 sets
Day 2 (LI)	4–6 sets	4–6 sets	5+ sets	5+ sets
Day 3 (TT/Endurance)	45–60 min	50–80 min	50–80 min	60–90 min
LAE (Chores, yard work, gardening, shoveling, etc.)	60–90 min	60–120 min	60–120 min	60–120 min

PRO

Warm-Up and Cooldown

Champions don't jump into training or competition without a warm-up and aren't done until after a cooldown and mobility work. So before and after each session, we suggest you follow this simple yet highly effective protocol. For more guidance on the breathing aspect, see powerspeedendurance.com, and check out www.mobilitywod.com and Kelly Starrett's book *Becoming a Supple Leopard,* second edition, for all the mobility exercises you'll ever need.

Warm-Up

1. 10 minutes nose-only breathing.

2. 5 minutes of 20 seconds progressively harder running, rowing, cycling, etc., followed by 40 seconds of easy (40 to 50 percent effort) activity. Try to make sure you breathe in through your nose and out through your mouth.

Cooldown

1. 5–10 minute walk (outdoors if possible) or easy nose-only breathing.

2. Mobility exercises on directly affected tissues (meaning those that feel tight, sore, or did the most work). As you're doing each mobilization, take a full breath in through your nose and hold for 3–5 seconds as you stay in the position. Then release and relax. Repeat for 2–3 minutes for each mobility exercise, or until you stop seeing positive changes, like increased range of motion or decreased pain or stiffness.

Take Your Training Off the Grid

Keep in mind one critical fact as you read this chapter: exercises do not determine adaptation, nor does the room in which you do them. Application determines adaptation. What I mean by this is that any of the workout routines listed above can be performed with virtually any exercise choice (or even a combination of several different movements), and in any environment you want. *How* you do the exercise (both the prescription—the number of reps, duration of the work period, rest intervals, etc.—and the technique with which you execute the exercise) determines the results you get, not the exercise itself. Cycling doesn't help you lose weight. Exercise does. Deadlifting doesn't make you strong. Moving heavy things does.

That's why we encourage you to have as much variation as possible in how you train and to be active outdoors as much as possible. If you take this training program and finish all sixteen

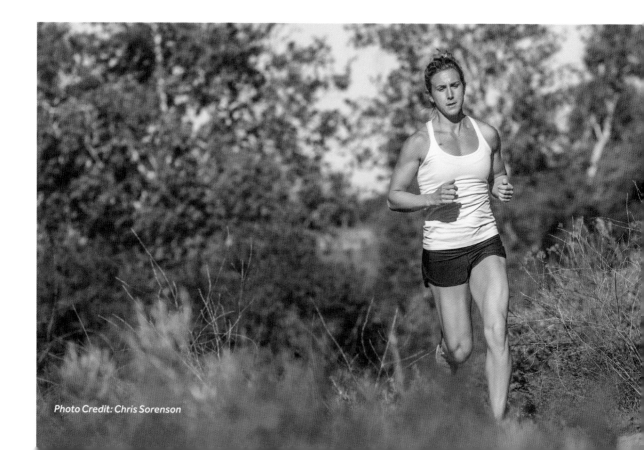

Photo Credit: Chris Sorenson

workouts (four times a week for four weeks) doing just one kind of exercise, like running on a treadmill or riding a spinning bike in your garage, you've missed the point of this book. Go back and start at page one! This is not to say that running on a treadmill or cycling at home is pointless or even bad for you. But we want you to take this training template and modify the details of execution based on your environment, experience level, geography, personal preferences, and equipment availability. We encourage you to get creative and introduce as much variety as you can. This is especially true if you're not engaging in a sport.

Say you're a city person who's loving life in the middle of a major urban metropolis like Dallas, Los Angeles, or Chicago. Getting access to nature might be difficult and fairly unrealistic during the work week. However, instead of just hitting the treadmill at your local tech-overloaded gym, a realistic compromise might look something like this:

Day 1	Do **SI** work with body weight movements (jumping jacks, burpees, etc.) in your front yard.
Day 2	Do **LI** work by running short hill sprints at the local park or a hilly neighborhood that's only a $6 Uber ride away.
Day 3	Do endurance work on an Airdyne or Assault AirBike at the local gym, in the basement of your building, or even in your house or apartment.
Day 4	Do **LAE** work by walking to your job, taking a cycling tour of the city, or hitting a skate park for an hour. This will not only get you outdoors but will also help you get to know your city better.

Every other weekend, try to take a day trip and exchange one of your "city workouts" for sprinting up and down the rolling hills, doing intervals of push-ups, air squats, hollow holds, and walking lunges at the base of a mountain, crushing a circuit training routine with a kettlebell in an open prairie, or doing intervals of dragging a log up and down the beach mixed with swimming or paddling.

However, if you're in a rural setting and training in nature is much more accessible, you could implement a simple routine like the following:

Day 1	Do **SI** sessions outside by using a combination of heavy dumbbell and barbell movements (or sandbags, dry bags filled with water, buckets filled with pebbles, or other low-budget accessories you could buy for a few dollars at your local hardware store).
Day 2	Do **LI** work by pushing a wheelbarrow or heavy sled or flipping an old tire through your field. If you live in a wooded area, you could also drag and flip logs.
Day 3	Do endurance work by swimming in the ocean or an outdoor pool, or by paddling in the sea or on a lake.
Day 4	Do **LAE** work by exploring new mountain biking or hiking trails, taking a long road bike session through the cornfields, or raking your leaves.

Regardless of whether you're in a city, the countryside, or somewhere in between, let go of your usual workout routine and allow your creativity to guide you. Why does your physical practice have to be boring and repetitive? It doesn't, if you build in some time for outdoor play. Don't let the weather in your area deter you either: these aren't summer-only options for being active outside. Why grind through a forty-five-minute elliptical LAE session in your garage when you could shovel snow from your driveway? Yes, I know you can pay someone forty dollars to mow and trim your lawn once a week, but why let them rob you of some stress-free, unstructured movement? Who says you can't replace your workout with taking your kids for a walk and having fun stomping in puddles?

Challenge Yourself

Listen to a few minutes of Dan Carlin's brilliant podcast *Hardcore History* and pay attention to the living conditions soldiers endured in the last century. You'll likely cringe with embarrassment at how fragile we've become when we can't handle the thought of going for a walk in the rain, knowing we have a warm house, digital dryer, and hot shower just minutes away.

The blinding speed and comfortableness of our technology age makes it hard to keep hardships in perspective, but extraordinary feats of survival were achieved by millions of people on a daily basis for years. And overcoming adversity isn't something that was only achieved by your "ancient hominid ancestors" (aka the Paleolithic forebears that certain fitness communities idolize), either. In fact, you likely know at least a few people who put themselves to the test on a regular basis.

That can be you, too. You might not be at the level of supreme natural movers like Ido Portal or Erwan Le Corre or explorers like Tim Jarvis yet (nor do you need to be), but anyone can begin cultivating practices to reconnect with their body and recalibrate their diminished senses. Maybe you start simply with a ten-day news and social media fast, ten hours of intermittent fasting (say from breakfast to dinner), or a ten-minute cool shower. Your physiology is meant to endure, so challenge it from time to time or you'll lose touch with it. (See Scott Carney's excellent book *What Doesn't Kill Us* for much more on this topic.) Apply your own creativity to these four basic principles:

1. Implement massive variety.
2. Use a combination of technology and unplugged activity, but do so with a purpose.
3. Integrate your training program with your *Unplugged* program (see page 238).
4. Apply the principles you've learned throughout this book to your life, exercise, and profession as much as possible and see if you feel the difference.

You can use the challenges in the table on page 253 to improve your internal calibration for basic sensations like hunger, heat, cold, fatigue, and thirst. Of course, do these at your own risk—under a physician's supervision if needed—progress slowly, and, most importantly, *listen to your body.*

Remember, trying to push yourself to failure is unnecessary. Instead, you should search for the first signs of an impending breakdown, like feeling dizzy when you're working out hard or shivering uncontrollably when you're cold. Note these, stop the experiment, and try to improve your tolerance the next time. More importantly, in that moment when you first notice the symptoms, aim to develop heightened awareness of your feelings and reactions. Are you really that hungry, or are you just uncomfortable because you're not used to going more than a couple of hours without food? Can you really feel the difference on days when you're fully hydrated and days you let it slide? For example, if you're five hours into the thirst challenge and you start feeling dizzy, stop what you're doing and really pay attention to your body. If it's screaming for water, get water. Challenge over! Next month try it again for five and a half hours. Or maybe you're thirsty and uncomfortable but in no real physical danger. Then perhaps press on for a few more hours, paying attention to any signs and symptoms.

Do not attempt any of these challenges while operating machinery, if you have a preexisting medical condition, or when other human lives are in your hands. However, I do recommend trying them on busy days, especially the challenges involving fasting and exposing yourself to hot and cold—having other things to do makes the time go faster and makes it easier to ignore any feelings of deprivation. You could combine several of these challenges at once, but again, be careful and smart. For example, you could do a twenty-four-hour fast while camping (fasting—check; unplugged—check; nature—check). However, don't add the fasting challenge if you've never camped before or are in an area you're unfamiliar with. Similarly, don't do the cold challenge by swimming in the ocean on a stormy day when no lifeguards are around. You definitely want a physical challenge, but there's no need to take unnecessary risks when the consequences could be life-threatening.

I routinely strap on snowshoes and explore the mountains of central Oregon without a map, food, much water, or thermal gear. (Indeed, Phil and I interviewed Tim Ferriss for this book while I was climbing a mountain with a friend.) However, I've been doing things like this for decades. Sure, the surfers I know drop into fifty-foot waves and make it seem effortless. But they spend each minute of every day preparing for such challenges and have decades of experience. While I truly believe you're capable of far more than you imagine, you don't need to take on the harshest environments on the planet or the most extreme self-challenges today. It's better to start with small steps, like a twelve-hour fast while doing some light yard work, taking a hot bath followed by a cold shower, or cutting the cord once a week. Remember, these challenges are not for stroking your ego. They are simply calibration tools that can help you live a better, more attuned, and more fully conscious life.

Unplugged Challenges

	BRONZE	SILVER	GOLD
HUNGER	16-hour fast once a month	24-hour fast once a month	48-hour fast once a month
CHEAT MEAL Absolutely no cheat meals (i.e., a day when you don't have any unhealthy meals)	1 week; once a quarter	2 weeks; 3 times per year	1 month; twice a year
HEAT Get really hot in a sauna, hot tub, or steam room; by wearing sweats while working out, etc.	Twice a month	Once a week	3 times per week
COLD Get really cold by taking a 2-minute cold shower, a 45-minute swim in the ocean, a one-minute ice bath, or a walk outside in a T-shirt in chilly conditions	Twice a month	Once a week	3 times per week
SLEEP 9+ hours a night	Once a week	6 times per month	10 times per month
FATIGUE Sleep less than 6 hours on back-to-back nights, or less than 10 hours total on 3 consecutive nights	Once a year	Once a quarter	Once every other month
HYDRATION Drink half of your body weight in pounds in fluid ounces of water a day, adding a pinch of sea salt to each glass to improve absorption	One day a quarter	1 week a month	2 weeks once a quarter
THIRST Go 12–24 hours without drinking any fluids	Once a year	Once a quarter	Once every other month
TECHNOLOGY UNPLUGGED Go 24 hours without any screen time (e-mail, social media, news, TV, etc.)	Once a month	Twice a month	40 times a year, or roughly 3.3 times a month
UNPLUG IN NATURE Spend 12+ hours in nature with little to no personal technology, outside of basic survival and safety equipment	2 days (cumulative) per quarter (8 days total per year)	4 days (cumulative) per quarter (16 days total per year)	7.5 days (cumulative) per quarter (30 days total per year)

Rocky or Drago?

If you asked moviegoers to name the best training montage in film history, I bet many would choose Rocky versus Drago from *Rocky IV*. Ivan Drago, played by Dolph Lundgren, is Rocky's opponent from the Soviet Union, and he takes the high-tech, ultramodern route for training for the big fight while working-class Philadelphia slugger Rocky goes super low-tech in Siberia. While Drago runs on a treadmill in the comfort of an air-conditioned building, Rocky tramps through a snow-covered, wind-whipped landscape. A team of Russian scientists monitors Drago's vital signs when raising the incline of his treadmill as Rocky struggles up a mountainside alone, relying on his instincts to take him to the summit. While Drago performs leg extensions and shoulder exercises on machines, Rocky helps a man pull his horse and buggy out of a frozen ditch. Drago cuts down sparring partners in the ring; Rocky chops down a tree with an axe. They might be developing the same muscles and energy systems, but who has the richer experience?

Drago is driven by steroids, human growth hormone, and the Soviet state's demands, while for Rocky, the clean mountain air and determination to defeat his nemesis are fuel enough. The Russian coaches time Drago's laps with a stopwatch and measure his exertion with a machine, urging him to run faster and lift heavier. Rocky pushes himself to exhaustion as he carries a log across his shoulders through a snowdrift, pulls his trainer on a sled like a Siberian husky, and heaves a giant bag of rocks off the ground.

Watch the clip on YouTube and tell me if you want to be Drago. No takers? That's because it's Rocky who inspires us. Beyond the Cold War patriotism and cheesy eighties music, his labors tap into something vital and elemental that we've buried beneath all the data we've collected, the artificial rewards we've earned, and the steps that we've counted. In our overconnected lives, we long to unplug and return to those same emotions Rocky experiences when he's fighting against his own limits and the Russian winter to reach a seemingly impossible goal.

Above all, we just want to feel again. And we're never going to get there while we're stuck in a gym, hooked on technology, and disconnected from nature, each other, and ourselves. Stop being Drago. Go out and be Rocky. Or better yet, be the best version of you. Unplug, get outside, and reconnect with your instincts. You'll be happier and healthier and will perform better for longer.

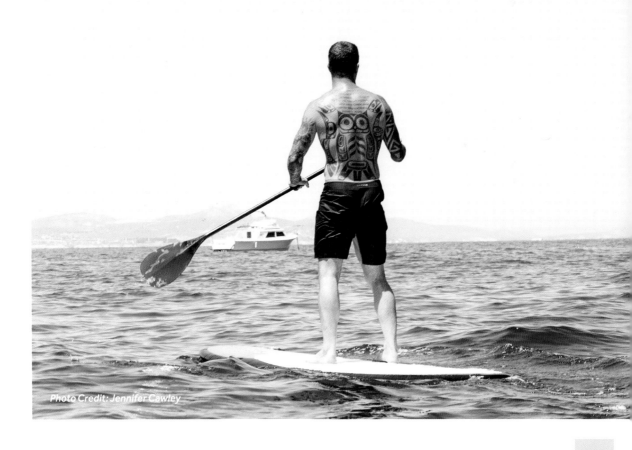

Photo Credit: Jennifer Cawley

SOURCES

Introduction

[1] Scott Adams, interview by Joe Rogan, *The Joe Rogan Experience*, November 17, 2016, http://podcasts.joerogan.net/podcasts/scott-adams.

[2] Laird Hamilton, interview with the author, January 30, 2017.

[3] Tim Ferriss, interview with the author, January 17, 2017.

[4] Julia Belluz and Sarah Frostenson, "Life Expectancy in the US Has Dropped for the First Time in Decades," *Vox*, December 8, 2016, http://www.vox.com/2016/12/8/13875150/life-expectancy-us-dropped-first-time-decade.

[5] Austin Frakt, "Blame Technology, Not Longer Life Spans, for Health Spending Increases," *New York Times*, January 23, 2017, https://www.nytimes.com/2017/01/23/upshot/blame-technology-not-longer-life-spans-for-health-spending-increases.html.

[6] Ericsson ConsumerLab, *Wearable Technology and the Internet of Things*, June 2016, https://www.ericsson.com/thinkingahead/consumerlab/consumer-insights/wearable-technology-and-the-internet-of-things.

[7] Rikke Duus and Mike Cooray, "Can Wearable Fitness Trackers Take Control of Your Life?," *Sydney Morning Herald*, June 22, 2015, http://www.smh.com.au/digital-life/wearables/can-wearable-fitness-trackers-take-control-of-your-life-20150622-ghumle.

[8] Amy Craft, "Fitbit Users Sue, Claiming Heart Rate Monitor Is Inaccurate," CBSNews.com, January 7, 2016, http://www.cbsnews.com/news/fitbit-users-sue-claiming-heart-rate-monitor-is-inaccurate.

[9] Kalyeena Makortoff, "Study Claims Fitbit Trackers Are 'Highly Inaccurate,'" CNBC.com, May 23, 2016, http://www.cnbc.com/2016/05/23/study-shows-fitbit-trackers-highly-inaccurate.html.

[10] Ferriss interview.

[11] Kai Lenny, interview with the author, January 23, 2017.

Chapter 1

[12] David Pierce, "Inside Fitbit's Quest to Make Fitness Trackers Invisible," *Wired*, August 2015; Nicholas Rossolillo, "Wearable Tech Has a World to Grow Into," *Fox Business*, December 10, 2016; Paul Lamkin, "Wearable Tech Market to Be

Worth $34 Billion by 2020," *Forbes*, February 2016, https://www.forbes.com/sites/paullamkin/2016/02/17/wearable-tech-market-to-be-worth-34-billion-by-2020/#3d9e6ea33cb5.

[13] Dan Diamond, "Just 8% of People Achieve Their New Year's Resolutions. Here's How They Do It," *Forbes*, January 1, 2013, http://www.forbes.com/sites/dandiamond/2013/01/01/just-8-of-people-achieve-their-new-years-resolutions-heres-how-they-did-it/#73492b8a304c.

[14] Anick Jesdanun, "Strong Sales, but High Abandonment for Fitness Trackers," *Associated Press*, July 9, 2015, http://bigstory.ap.org/article/2700956044de4517a471a47c3243078b/strong-sales-high-abandonment-fitness-trackers.

[15] Dr. Susan Weinschenk, "Why We're All Addicted to Texts, Twitter and Google," *Psychology Today*, September 11, 2012, https://www.psychologytoday.com/blog/brain-wise/201209/why-were-all-addicted-texts-twitter-and-google.

[16] Cari Romm, "The Nihilistic Angst of Quitting Your Fitbit," *New York Magazine*, August 26, 2016, http://nymag.com/scienceofus/2016/08/i-quit-fitbit-and-fell-into-nihilistic-despair.html.

[17] Rose Eveleth, "Academics Write Papers Arguing over How Many People Read (and Cite) Their Papers," *Smithsonian*, March 25, 2014, http://www.smithsonianmag.com/smart-news/half-academic-studies-are-never-read-more-three-people-180950222/#w4J9O9Kq7B2O2wbg.99.

[18] Anahad O'Connor, "For Coffee Drinkers, the Buzz May Be in Your Genes," *New York Times*, July 12, 2016, http://well.blogs.nytimes.com/2016/07/12/for-coffee-drinkers-the-buzz-may-be-in-your-genes.

[19] James A. Woodman et al., "Accuracy of Consumer Monitors for Estimating Energy Expenditure and Activity Type," *Medicine and Science in Sport and Exercise* 49, no. 2 (February 2017), doi: 10.1249/MSS.0000000000001090.

[20] Stacey Colino, "Do Exercise Machines Lie? What You Need to Know About the Feedback You Get," *US News and World Report*, December 15, 2015, http://health.usnews.com/health-news/health-wellness/articles/2015-12-23/do-exercise-machines-lie-what-you-need-to-know-about-the-feedback-you-get.

[21] Charles M. Tipton, ed., *History of Exercise Physiology* (Champaign, IL: Human Kinetics, 2014).

[22] G. Edgar Folk, "The Harvard Fatigue Laboratory Brought Aid and Comfort to America's WWII GIs" (press release), American Physiological Society, September 13, 2010, http://www.the-aps.org/mm/hp/Audiences/Public-Press/Archive/2010/28.html.

[23] Martin Miller, "The Standard Heart Rate Formula Might Be an Exercise in Futility," *Chicago Tribune*, April 13, 2003, http://articles.chicagotribune.com/2003-04-13/features/0304130155_1_formula-underwent-numerous-revisions-maximum-heart-rate-formula-maximum-heart.

24 Robert A. Robergs and Roberto Landwehr, "The Surprising History of the 'HRmax=220–Age' Equation," *Journal of Exercise Physiology* 5, no. 2 (May 2002), https://www.asep.org/asep/asep/Robergs2.pdf.

25 Scott Trappe et al., "New Records in Aerobic Power Among Octogenarian Lifelong Endurance Athletes," *Journal of Applied Physiology* 114 (October 2012), doi: 10.1152/japplphysiol.01107.2012.

26 K. F. Koltyn and W. P. Morgan, "Efficacy of Perceptual Versus Heart Rate Monitoring in the Development of Endurance," *British Journal of Sports Medicine* 26, no. 2 (1992), http://europepmc.org/backend/ptpmcrender.fcgi?accid=PMC1478928&blobtype=pdf.

27 Ferriss interview.

28 Ibid.

29 A. E. Sleigh et al., "Efficacy of Tart Cherry Juice to Reduce Inflammation Among Patients with Osteoarthritis," presentation at the annual meeting of the American College of Sports Medicine, San Francisco, California, May 30, 2012.

30 Jon-Philippe K. Hyatt et al., "Muscle-Specific Myosin Heavy Chain Shifts in Response to a Long-Term High Fat / High Sugar Diet and Resveratrol Treatment in Nonhuman Primates," *Frontiers in Physiology* 7, no. 77 (March 2016), doi: 10.3389/fphys.2016.00077.

31 R. L. Rankin et al., "Test-Retest Reliability and Validity of the 400-Meter Walk Test in Healthy, Middle-Aged Women," *Journal of Physical Activity and Health* 7, no. 5 (September 2010), https://www.ncbi.nlm.nih.gov/pubmed/20864761; Jamie F. Burr et al., "The 6-Minute Walk Test as a Predictor of Objectively Measured Aerobic Fitness in Healthy Working-Aged Adults," *The Physician and Sportsmedicine* 39, no. 2 (May 2011), doi: 10.3810/psm.2011.05.1904.

32 Tom Haberstroh, "Sources: NBA, Players Plan to Form Wearables Committee as Part of New CBA," ESPN.com, December 14, 2016, http://www.espn.com/nba/story/_/id/18281782/nba-players-plan-form-new-wearables-committee-part-new-cba.

33 Kathryn C. Montgomery, Jeff Chester, and Katharina Kopp, *Health Wearable Devices in the Big Data Era: Ensuring Privacy, Security, and Consumer Protection*, Center for Digital Democracy, American University, December 15, 2016, https://www.democraticmedia.org/sites/default/files/field/public/2016/aucdd_wearablesreport_final121516.pdf.

34 Ibid.

35 "Your Medical Records," US Department of Health and Human Services, https://www.hhs.gov/hipaa/for-individuals/medical-records.

36 "Individual Access to Medical Records: 50 State Comparison," Hirsh Health Law and Policy Program, George Washington University, and the Robert Wood Johnson Foundation, http://www.healthinfolaw.org/comparative-analysis/individual-access-medical-records-50-state-comparison.

37 Emma Poole, "The Brave New World of Wearable Technology: What Implications for IP?," *WIPO Magazine*, http://www.wipo.int/wipo_magazine/en/2014/03/article_0002.html.

38 Sarah O'Connor, "Wearables at Work: The New Frontier of Employee Surveillance," *Financial Times*, June 8, 2015, https://www.ft.com/content/d7eee768-0b65-11e5-994d-00144feabdc0.

39 Olivia Solon, "Wearable Technology Creeps into the Workplace," *Bloomberg*, August 6, 2015, https://www.bloomberg.com/news/articles/2015-08-07/wearable-technology-creeps-into-the-workplace.

40 Siraj Datoo, "These Companies Are Tracking the Fitness of Their Employees," *The Guardian*, March 17, 2014, https://www.theguardian.com/technology/2014/mar/17/why-companies-are-tracking-the-fitness-of-their-employees.

41 O'Connor, "Wearables at Work."

42 Sarah O'Connor, interview by Renee Montagne, "Are You Willing to Share Your Wearables Data with Your Boss?," *Morning Edition*, NPR, June 2, 2015, http://www.npr.org/2015/06/02/411406418/are-you-willing-to-share-your-wearables-technology-data-with-your-boss.

43 Ibid.

44 Jad Abumrad and Robert Krulwich, "Colors," *Radiolab*, May 21, 2012, http://www.radiolab.org/story/211119-colors.

Chapter 2

45 Catherine Shanahan, MD, with Luke Shanahan, *Deep Nutrition: Why Your Genes Need Traditional Food* (New York, NY: Flatiron Books, 2016), xvii.

46 Ibid., xviii.

47 Adam Alter, *Irresistible: The Rise of Addictive Technology and the Business of Keeping Us Hooked* (New York, NY: Penguin, 2017), 113.

48 "Facebook Status Updates Reveal Low Self-Esteem and Narcissism," Brunel University London, May 22, 2015, http://www.brunel.ac.uk/news-and-events/news/articles/Facebook-status-updates-reveal-low-self-esteem-and-narcissism.

49 Hamilton interview, January 30, 2017.

50 Laird Hamilton, interview with the author, January 17, 2017.

51 Jeff Foss, "The Tale of a Fitness Tracking Addict's Struggles with Strava," *Wired*, October 3, 2014, https://www.wired.com/2014/10/my-strava-problem.

52 Sherry Page et al., "The Weight Loss Blogosphere: An Online Survey of Weight Loss Bloggers," *Translational Behavioral Medicine* 6, no. 3 (September 2016), https://www.ncbi.nlm.nih.gov/pubmed/27528529.

53 Brad Stulberg, "Fitness Trackers Fail Because They're Not Human," *Outside*, December 27, 2016, https://www.outsideonline.com/2143956/fitness-trackers-fail-because-theyre-not-human.

54 Frank Merritt, interview with the author, December 20, 2016.

55 Michael Winnick, "Putting a Finger on Our Phone Obsession," *DScout*, June 16, 2016, https://blog.dscout.com/mobile-touches.

56 Mark W. Smith, "A Fitbit Fanatic's Cry for Help," *Washington Post*, May 11, 2015, https://www.washingtonpost.com/news/to-your-health/wp/2015/05/11/a-fitbit-fanatics-cry-for-help.

57 Nora Krug, "Is Technology Spoiling Your Workout?" *Washington Post*, March 10, 2015, https://www.washingtonpost.com/lifestyle/wellness/is-technology-spoiling-your-workout/2015/03/09/3a7cb6bc-c02f-11e4-ad5c-3b8ce89f1b89_story.html.

58 Foss, "The Tale of a Fitness Tracking Addict's Struggles with Strava."

59 Romm, "The Nihilistic Angst of Quitting Your Fitbit."

60 Lenny Wiersma, interview with the author.

61 Dave Asprey, *Head Strong: The Bulletproof Plan to Activate Untapped Brain Energy to Work Smarter and Think Faster—in Just Two Weeks* (New York, NY: Harper Wave, 2017), 9.

62 Jon Mooallem, "Don't Wear a Fitbit Just Because Your Partner Says So," *Wired*, March 9, 2017, https://www.wired.com/2017/03/mr-know-it-all-12.

63 Howard Tullman, "Fitbit Anxiety Is Part of a Larger Problem," *Inc.*, July 1, 2014, http://www.inc.com/howard-tullman/fitbit-anxiety-is-part-of-a-larger-problem.html.

64 Wiersma interview.

65 Tim Ferriss, *Tools of Titans: The Tactics, Routines, and Habits of Billionaires, Icons, and World-Class Performers* (New York: Houghton Mifflin Harcourt, 2017), 412.

Chapter 3

66 Linda Stone, "Continuous Partial Attention," https://lindastone.net/qa/continuous-partial-attention/.

67 Robert Sapolsky, *Why Zebras Don't Get Ulcers* (New York: Henry Holt and Company, 1994), 48.

68 Ibid.

69 Frank Merritt, interview with the author, December 8, 2016.

70 Wiersma interview.

[71] Robert Greene, *Mastery* (New York: Penguin, 2012), 77.

[72] Saubarh S. Thosar et al., "Effect of Prolonged Sitting and Breaks in Sitting Time on Endothelial Function," *Medicine and Science in Sports and Exercise* 47, no. 4 (April 2015), http://journals.lww.com/acsm-msse/Citation/2015/04000/Effect_of_Prolonged_Sitting_and_Breaks_in_Sitting.22.aspx.

[73] Gregory Garrett et al., "Call Center Productivity Over 6 Months Following a Standing Desk Intervention," *IIE Transactions on Occupational Ergonomics and Human Factors* 4, no. 2–3 (April 2016), doi: 10.1080/21577323.2016.1183534.

[74] Richard P. Dum, David J. Levinthal, and Peter L. Strick, "Motor, Cognitive, and Affective Areas of the Cerebral Cortex Influence the Adrenal Medulla," *Proceedings of the National Academy of Sciences of the United States* 113, no. 35 (July 2016), http://www.pnas.org/content/113/35/9922.abstract.

[75] Gretchen Reynolds, "Keep It Moving," *New York Times,* December 9, 2016, www.nytimes.com/2016/12/09/well/move/keep-it-moving.html.

Chapter 4

[76] Neil Kleipis et al., "The National Human Activity Pattern Survey (NHAPS): A Resource for Assessing Exposure to Environmental Pollutants," *Journal of Exposure Science and Environmental Epidemiology* 11 (2001), http://www.nature.com/jes/journal/v11/n3/full/7500165a.html.

[77] Lenny interview.

[78] Ibid.

[79] "5 Benefits of Houseplants," Learning Center, Bayer, https://www.bayeradvanced.com/articles/5-benefits-of-houseplants.

[80] Jacqueline Howard, "Americans Devote More Than 10 Hours a Day to Screen Time, and Growing," *Time*, July 29, 2016, http://www.cnn.com/2016/06/30/health/americans-screen-time-nielsen.

[81] Lenny interview.

[82] Ruth Anne Kocour, *Facing the Extreme: One Woman's Tale of True Courage, Death-Defying Survival, and Her Quest for the Summit* (New York: St. Martin's Press, 1998), 5.

[83] Lenny interview.

[84] Jessica de Bloom et al., "Vacation (After-) Effects on Employee Health and Well-Being, and the Role of Vacation Activities, Experiences and Sleep," *Journal of Happiness Studies* 14, no. 2 (April 2013), http://link.springer.com/article/10.1007/s10902-012-9345-3.

[85] Florence Williams, "This Is Your Brain on Nature," *National Geographic*, January 2016, http://ngm.nationalgeographic.com/2016/01/call-to-wild-text.

86 Olga Khazan, "How Walking in Nature Prevents Depression," *The Atlantic*, June 30, 2015, http://www.theatlantic.com/health/archive/2015/06/how-walking-in-nature-prevents-depression/397172.

87 Shilo Rea, "Mental Maps: Route Learning Changes Brain Tissue," *CMU News*, October 27, 2015, http://www.cmu.edu/news/stories/archives/2015/october/mental-maps.html.

88 Joseph Hooper, "The Radical Calm of Alex Honnold," *Men's Journal,* September 2015, http://www.mensjournal.com/magazine/the-radical-calm-of-alex-honnold-20150908.

89 Kevin Rushby, "Climber Tommy Caldwell: 'From an Early Age Yosemite Became the Center of My Universe,'" *The Telegraph,* November 27, 2015, https://www.theguardian.com/travel/2015/nov/27/yosemite-climber-tommy-caldwell-el-capitan-dawn-wall.

90 Hooper, "The Radical Calm of Alex Honnold."

91 Frank Merritt, interview with the author, December 6, 2016.

92 Ibid.

93 Wiersma interview.

94 Lenny interview.

95 Ibid.

96 Ibid.

Chapter 5

97 Larry Rosen, *iDisorder: Understanding Our Obsession with Technology and Overcoming Its Hold on Us* (New York, NY: St. Martin's Press, 2012), 5.

98 Hamilton interview, January 31, 2017.

99 Mick Cleary, "England Players Told Mobile Phones Are Bad for Their Game by Vision Consultant Sherylle Calder," *The Telegraph*, January 23, 2017, http://www.telegraph.co.uk/rugby-union/2017/01/23/england-players-told-mobile-phones-bad-game-vision-consultantsherylle.

100 Wiersma interview.

101 Lenny interview.

102 Erin Cafaro-Mackenzie, interview with the author.

103 Wiersma interview.

Chapter 6

104 "Adult Obesity Facts," Centers for Disease Control and Prevention, https://www.cdc.gov/obesity/data/adult.html.

105 John M. Jakicic et al., "Effect of Wearable Technology Combined with a Lifestyle Intervention on Long-Term Weight Loss: The IDEA Randomized Clinical Trial," *JAMA* 316, no. 11 (September 20, 2016), http://jamanetwork.com/journals/jama/article-abstract/2553448.

106 Nicole Avena, "Your Fitbit Is Ruining Your Relationship with Your Body," *Psychology Today,* September 28, 2015, https://www.psychologytoday.com/blog/food-junkie/201509/your-fitbit-is-ruining-your-relationship-your-body.

107 M. Wei et al., "Relationship Between Low Cardiorespiratory Fitness and Mortality in Normal-Weight, Overweight, and Obese Men," *JAMA* 282, no. 16 (1999), https://www.ncbi.nlm.nih.gov/pubmed/10546694.

108 D. P. Leong, "Prognostic Value of Grip Strength: Findings from the Prospective Urban Rural Epidemiology (PURE) Study," *The Lancet* 386, no. 9990 (July 2015), http://www.thelancet.com/journals/lancet/article/PIIS0140-6736(14)62000-6/abstract.

109 Frank Merritt, interview with the author, December 16, 2016.

110 Michael Lewis, *The Blind Side: Evolution of a Game* (New York, NY: W. W. Norton, 2007), 225.

111 Merritt interview, December 16, 2016.

112 Hamilton interview, January 30, 2017.

Chapter 7

113 Bob Bowman, *The Golden Rules: 10 Steps to World-Class Excellence in Your Life and Work*, 13.

114 Wiersma interview.

115 Ferriss interview.

116 Cafaro-Mackenzie interview.

117 Lindsey Crouse, "His Strength Sapped, Top Marathoner Ryan Hall Decides to Stop," *New York Times*, January 15, 2016, http://www.nytimes.com/2016/01/17/sports/ryan-hall-fastest-us-distance-runner-is-retiring.html.

118 Erin Strout, "That's Not Fat: How Ryan Hall Gained 40 Pounds of Muscle," *Runner's World*, May 3, 2016, http://www.runnersworld.com/elite-runners/thats-not-fat-how-ryan-hall-gained-40-pounds-of-muscle.

Chapter 8

[119] Rikke Duus and Michael Cooray, "How We Discovered the Dark Side of Wearable Fitness Trackers," *The Conversation*, June 19, 2015, http://theconversation. com/how-we-discovered-the-dark-side-of-wearable-fitness-trackers-43363.

[120] Dom D'Agostino, interview by Tim Ferriss, "Dom D'Agostino—The Power of the Ketogenic Diet," *The Tim Ferris Podcast,* July 2016, http://fourhourworkweek. com/2016/07/06/dom-dagostino-part-2; W. K. Stewart and Laura W. Fleming, "Features of a Successful Therapeutic Fast of 382 Days' Duration," *Postgraduate Medical Journal* 49, no. 569 (March 1973), https://www.ncbi. nlm.nih.gov/pmc/articles/PMC2495396/.

[121] Chiara Milanese et al., "The Effects of Two Different Correction Strategies on the Snatch Technique in Weightlifting," *Journal of Sports Sciences* 35, no. 5 (2017), http://www.tandfonline.com/doi/abs/10.1080/02640414.2016.1172727.

[122] Hamilton interview, January 30, 2017.

[123] Wiersma interview.

[124] Jordan Etkin, "The Hidden Cost of Personal Quantification," *Journal of Consumer Research* 42, no. 6 (February 16, 2016), http://jcr.oxfordjournals.org/content/ early/2016/02/16/jcr.ucv095.

[125] Hamilton interview, January 30, 2017.

Chapter 9

[126] Tim Ferriss, *The 4-Hour Body: An Uncommon Guide to Rapid Fat-Loss, Incredible Sex, and Becoming Superhuman* (New York: Crown Archetype, 2010), 4.

[127] Thich Nhat Hanh, *The Miracle of Mindfulness: An Introduction to the Practice of Meditation* (Boston: Beacon Press, 1975), 5.

[128] Maggie Fox, "One in 6 Americans Take Antidepressants, Other Psychiatric Drugs: Study," NBCNews.com, December 12, 2016, http://www.nbcnews. com/health/health-news/one-6-americans-take-antidepressants-other-psychiatric-drugs-n695141; "PTSD Statistics," PTSD United, http://www. ptsdunited.org/ptsd-statistics-2.

[129] Steven Kotler, *The Rise of Superman* (Amazon Publishing, 2014).

[130] "The Science of Neuropriming," Halo Neuroscience, https://www.haloneuro. com/science.

INDEX

ABOUT THE AUTHORS

Brian Mackenzie is a world-renowned strength and conditioning expert and the author of the *New York Times* bestseller *Unbreakable Runner.* He is the founder of the training program Power Speed Endurance and the cofounder of the complete fitness lifestyle system XPT Life. Mackenzie has been featured in *Runner's World, Men's Journal, The Economist,* Tim Ferriss's *New York Times* bestseller *The 4-Hour Body*, and many other leading publications. Brian works with several CrossFit Games athletes, including champions Rich Froning Jr. and Annie Thorisdottir, and has guided world and Olympic champions and performance innovators like Laird Hamilton, Taylor Ritzel, Sara Hendershot, Jamie Mitchell, Koa Rothman, Koa and Alex Smith, Nathan Florence, and Elliot Sloan.

Dr. Andy Galpin is a professor of kinesiology at the Center for Sport Performance at California State University, Fullerton. He has a PhD in human bioenergetics and is the founder and director of the Biochemistry and Molecular Exercise Laboratory. Galpin works directly with professional athletes in the NFL, MLB, and UFC and played a major role in Helen Maroulis's run to gold in wrestling at the 2016 Rio Olympics. He is a cohost of the popular training podcast *Barbell Shrugged,* which has more than 300,000 followers, and has been featured in countless magazine articles, television shows, and other podcasts. One interviewer called him "the Tony Stark of human performance."

Phil White is an Emmy-nominated writer and the coauthor of *Waterman 2.0* and *Flight Plan* with Dr. Kelly Starrett. He also contributes to *The Inertia, SUP the Mag*, and *Canoe & Kayak.*